# ANAESTHESIA
# IN THE ELDERLY

# ANAESTHESIA IN THE ELDERLY

## HAROLD T. DAVENPORT

MB, ChB, FRCP(C), FFARCS(ENG.)

CONSULTANT ANAESTHETIST,
NORTHWICK PARK HOSPITAL AND CLINICAL RESEARCH CENTRE,
HARROW, ENGLAND

FORMERLY DIRECTOR OF ANAESTHESIA,
MONTREAL AND VANCOUVER CHILDREN'S HOSPITALS,
CANADA

## ELSEVIER
New York · Amsterdam · Oxford

*Elsevier Science Publishing Co., Inc.*
*52 Vanderbilt Avenue, New York,*
*New York 10017*

*Sole distributors outside the*
*United States and Canada:*

*William Heinemann Medical Books*
*23 Bedford Square, London WC1B 3HH*

ISBN 0–444–01047–5

PRINTED IN GREAT BRITAIN

# Contents

# Foreword

Dr Davenport has done me the great honour of asking me to write a foreword to this book. As a friend of some thirty years this is not difficult for me since I know him and his work very well indeed, and I regard the task as one of conveying some of this knowledge to the reader. It may seem strange to some, that one who has a world-wide reputation in paediatrics and paediatric anaesthesia, one who has written widely in that field and who has already published an excellent book on paediatric anaesthesia, should, at this late stage in his career turn to the subject of anaesthesia in the elderly. It is not at all strange to me because whatever Dr Davenport does in life is done well and is subjected to a keenly critical look. His work at Northwick Park Hospital involves much to do with the elderly patient, both in surgery and in the pain-relief clinic which he runs. He is endowed with the clear perception that all is not what it seems to be even although it is established practice.

Dr Davenport has carried out research wherever he has worked and a most impressive bibliography has accrued to his credit, his collaborators coming from many walks of medical life. It is not then surprising that one who is so keenly perceptive, so hard-working and so devoted a communicator should see the need for a textbook devoted to anaesthesia in the elderly. The text is packed with tightly condensed information, sifted and evaluated and presented to the reader in a typically clear style. It is not a book which can be skipped over quickly but one in which each page engages thought, stimulates enquiry and gives considered views from the literature and from Dr Davenport's own experience.

It is indeed a delight to read a single author book written in

this beautifully concise style with none of the salient features
˚obscured by padding, repetition or by an inability to say exactly
what is meant. A most useful and interesting book is here for
your information and delectation.


Sir Gordon Robson, CBE, (1986)

# Preface

There shall be no more thence an infant of days, nor an old man
that hath not filled his days; for the child shall die at a hundred
years old

*Isaiah 65: 20*

THE branch of medicine dealing with diseases of old age was
given the name 'geriatrics' by Dr I. Nascher (1914) of New
York 72 years ago. Unfortunately the word has now acquired
a connotation which is derogatory or depressive. By using the
word 'elderly' instead of 'geriatric' I hope that anaesthetists
will be alerted to the challenges and rewards of work in this
expanding field. The forms of anaesthesia for all humans are
similar, but we especially need to know the peculiarities of
treatment for the young and the old. It is now accepted that
an infant is not a miniature adult, and we should similarly
accept that an aged person is not a degenerate, feeble adult.
Both the young and the old differ from the mature person;
they have different anatomy, physiology, biochemistry and
psychology, and with such differences they must need different medicine, surgery and anaesthesia. Too much of the
anaesthesia for older patients has been undertaken by those
with limited experience and in emergency situations. A
patient over 75 years old requires medical expertise comparable to that provided for a neonate. Mismanagement of the
young can be disastrous, but mismanagement of the elderly is
more often fatal; in the latter case, however, we are unfortunately liable to be less conscience-stricken or medico-legally at
risk.

A recent British report on mortality (Lunn and Mushin,
1982) associated with anaesthesia stated that 'old age is
sometimes used to excuse a death', that 'anaesthetists regard
old age as a factor in determining death which cannot be
minimized by them' and 'they are more inclined to allocate
aged patients less often to the group in which anaesthesia is
totally responsible for a death'. Half of all patients over 65
years old have an operation before they die, and in my

lifetime the number of those over 65 has trebled, so such statements must cause us concern. The World Assembly on Ageing held by the United Nations in Austria in 1982 made the following statement with which I concur: 'support to the aged people must be provided by practitioners who are knowledgable in the subject of ageing, are interested in ageing people and their families, and are skilled in working with them and are concerned about the quality of care given.'

This book covers the practical aspects of anaesthesia management which are likely to influence the standard of care of the elderly. It has been written with the expectation that the reader will already have knowledge and experience of anaesthesia for mature patients. The subjects dealt with are those which I believe have not received sufficient attention or are not taught widely enough. Some important features are not detailed, for example the placement of central venous or arterial catheters, because they are adequately dealt with elsewhere. Chapters on the biology of older patients, and on their medical and surgical peculiarities, are presented with emphasis on matters of interest to anaesthetists. The remaining chapters and appendices are intended to broaden the understanding of the anaesthetists' contribution to work with the elderly, and will, it is hoped, encourage a much needed increase in research on the subject.

The references from English language publications, listed by chapter and subject, are not all-inclusive but are used as sources of facts or to complement my opinions in the construction of the text.

I would like to thank Gillian Oliver, Dr Eileen Twomey and the staff of the Department of Medical Illustration in the Clinical Research Centre, for the figures; also Jill Ainsworth, Ella Liddell and my wife, Margaret, for typing the many drafts of the manuscript. I am also grateful to Mr John Lewis, Dr Michael Denham and Dr Tony Coleman for their advice and to the staff of William Heinemann Medical Books for their indispensable assistance. Professor Sir Gordon Robson has very kindly contributed a foreword.

Harold T. Davenport
1986

**References**

Nascher I. R. (1914). *Geriatrics: The Diseases of Old Age and Their Treatment*. Philadelphia: Blakistons Son and Co.
Lunn J. N., Mushin W. W. (1982). Mortality associated with anaesthesia. London: *Nuffield Provincial Hospital Trust*.

# CHAPTER 1

# The elderly patient

*Every man desires to live long, but no man would be old.*
*Jonathan Swift*

## Introduction

The age limits of the 'young', 'mature' and 'old' are arbitrary. Commonly, those who are in retirement or pensionable (more than 60 or 65 years old) are called aged—except by those who are themselves that old! In the developed countries 15% of the population is over 60 years old, and it is usual for over twice that percentage of surgical beds to be occupied by patients of this age group. By the end of the century one in five persons in the U.K. will be over 60 because of the continued increase of the average life expectancy. The present pattern of age distribution in the newly developing countries is similar to that of Victorian England. Doubtless the pattern of change in developing countries will follow that of the developed countries, although it may be more rapid if there is zero growth rate of population and improved medical care. The reduction in the death rate of younger people has been apparent throughout history (Fig. 1.1), but preparation for the consequent changes in society has been given insufficient consideration.

If an anaesthetist is to encompass this growing need for medicine for the elderly, he or she has to understand the attitudes and aims of the specialists interested in the care of old people. The British pioneers in this field rejected the idea that chronic incurability was the norm in old patients, or that ageing constitutes an illness. Dr Marjory Warren, in London, created the first geriatric unit, with access to all the services of a general hospital, with the intention of curing old patients of the multiple diseases to which they are prone. It is in keeping with her philosophy that I would recommend the following measures in the care of the elderly.

The greatest feasible amount of day and home care should be used and hospital admission should be limited as far as possible. If admission is unavoidable, however, a colourful,

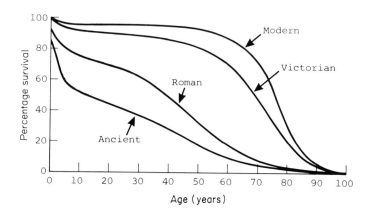

**Fig. 1.1** The increasingly rectangular survival curve throughout history with compression of the 'period of morbidity'.

stimulating decor will help patients to adjust to the hospital and will enable them to recognise and associate themselves easily with a particular ward. Lighting and heating should be well controlled. Adjustable beds, walking frames, lifting devices and adaptation for the ablutions of the disabled are all essential (Fig. 1.2). Administrative and visiting restrictions should be kept to the minimum. Extra precautions are required so that falls, electric shocks, scalds and other such accidents can be reduced as far as possible. By far the majority of accidents in hospital involve patients who are elderly (mean age 70 years).

Safety, feeding, nursing and occupational needs are best served by an adequate number of trained staff. But the staff-to-patient ratio is often too low. The present general nursing provision for geriatrics in Britain is, at best, 1 nurse to 1.8 patients, whereas the British Medical Association request was for 1:1.25 (without training commitment). The proportion of beds provided for those over 65 years old (which is still quite variable in general hospitals) should also be increased if we are to achieve the aims of Dr Warren.

## Psychology

The process of ageing can be said to comprise the less efficient regeneration of cells which follows the accomplish-

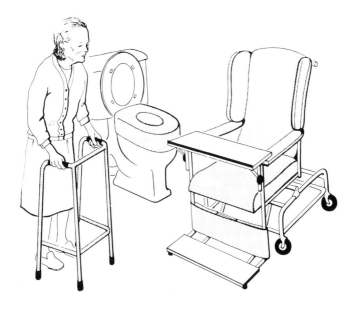

**Fig. 1.2** Three essential aids required for the use of elderly patients (a walking frame, a raised toilet and an adapted chair).

ment of full maturity. The brain is, however, not a regenerating but a finite organ. Changes in intellect in old age follow a pattern, with perceptual–interpretative ability, recent recollection, and skills requiring speed first affected. There is frequently a loss of ability to retain a memory of short-term experiences and it is this loss of recent memory that makes the mastery of facts for decision making difficult. Aphasia and deafness (which are 'normal') can make communication slow. The resultant difficulties which the elderly have in understanding new ideas and making decisions require patience on the part of those caring for them. Thus a consent form for an operation may need to be presented without haste, and perhaps repeatedly, before an elderly patient can sign it willingly. Confirming symptoms and eliciting signs are not as easy with the elderly, and a great deal of patience is called for, because these processes may be vital to the conduct of anaesthesia.

The old, as all of us, often respond better to direct contact from those offering help than to officious off-handedness. Every care must be taken to minimise any stress which may invade the structure of thought and disintegrate the mind's order. This, psychologists believe, causes defects of memory, awareness, orientation and intellectual functions in half the old patients admitted to hospital for operations under anaesthesia. The old are often insecure, and their daily surroundings seem unfriendly to them. They may therefore welcome illness and may prolong it as a means of being noticed and cared for properly. Their excessive restlessness and physical activity or quarrelsomeness may be due to chronic underactivity of the brain. The disengagement of the aged from and by society leads to a lack of spontaneity in their reaction to incidents. They take longer to adapt, do not like change, and need more time to learn about anything new.

The ageing mind is nevertheless resilient in the face of psychic trauma. The psychic pattern of the old varies with their physiological decline, and it is personality which is all important in adapting to change. It is quite unpardonable to use derogatory terms when referring to old patients, or to treat them as though they were in a second childhood. The caution and the suspicion that they exhibit often arise from adverse experiences, and a clear explanation will rarely be rejected, and will usually lead to cooperation and reason.

For the old, disease is not extraneous or viewed as a condition to be fought against, but rather an event which advances and announces the end of life. Illness can at first overwhelm them and precipitate a death wish, but even a minor improvement in their health will often dispel depression and activate the mainspring of their recovery—the desire to live.

## Examination

The process of ageing is a continuous biological change, now being extensively studied in the science of gerontology. We do not know the reasons for these natural changes with time, but theories abound (see Appendix A). An anaesthetist must understand the anatomical and physiological changes which occur in the elderly subject, and should be able to recognise their importance in his work. The number of active parenchymal cells decreases with age, and there is a concomitant increase of inactive interstitial cells. This is most obvious in tissues which divide and replace poorly, for example those of the kidney, nerves and muscles. The linear decline of a variety of physiological functions is at the yearly rate of 0.7–0.9% of capacity at 30 years old. Furthermore, there is the added complication of pathological degenerative states, such as arteriosclerosis and osteoporosis, which occur frequently, but are not exclusive to, or inevitable, in the elderly. Diseases of the old are more likely to be multiple, and they have a different pattern and invoke an altered response to those expected in younger patients. The need to obtain details of the history and home conditions of the patient indirectly from a guardian is comparable to that in paediatric practice, but it is also necessary to be aware of the tendency to minimise or not mention illness, as it is considered to be inevitable in the elderly.

## Appearance

We all become shorter as we age. The vertebral discs and bodies shrink. There is increased kyphosis and some degree of flexion of the hips and knees. There is bowing of the long bones of the legs, but the arms are unchanged in length. A young adult is usually slightly taller than his span measurement, but this is progressively reversed by ageing. At 60 years old the height and span are approximately equal, and at 90 years old the span measurement is an average of 8 cm greater than the height. The muscle size and average skinfold measurements decrease markedly in the lifetime of men, but less so in that of women. In all, the percentage of body weight due to fat tends to increase with ageing. However, the manner of distribution of subcutaneous fat changes, and forearm fat depots atrophy, even in those who are overweight. The breasts of women (gland and envelope), atrophy and hang lower. A decrease in subcutaneous fat means contours sharpen and hollows deepen. Bony landmarks, with muscle shapes and attachments, become more prominent and the axillary and intercostal spaces are excavated. Overall weight is usually reduced with ageing, so that fewer than 10% of the aged are overweight and more than 50% are underweight.

Skin everywhere becomes more fragile and dried, with an

anaemic look due to the loss of capillaries. However, grafts of old and young skin are equally vigorous. Brown pigmentation, especially of the exposed areas, causes senile freckles (or lentigo), which is clinically insignificant. The tendency for aged skin to bruise and form suction blisters easily may embarrass an anaesthetist. Repeated use of the muscles of expression, loss of fat and elastic tissue, and a lax skin lead to progressive facial wrinkling. This starts around the eyes, even in the 20s and at 60 fine crevices radiate round the mouth. Once the patient is toothless, reabsorption of the maxilla or mandible causes withering of the lower face. However, orbital bags and double chins do recede with old age.

## The nervous system

From about the age of 25, it is said that many brain and spinal cord cells die each day and that they are not replaced, but whether or not there is a significant ageing neuronal fallout is disputed. New automated cell counting shows reduced numbers of Purkinje cells in the cerebellum and of neurons in the locus coeruleus; however, with approximately 20 000 million cerebral neurons in each human, the reserve is unquestionable. Normally the brain is heaviest at about 17 years of age and weighs approximately 7% less at age 70. It is generally agreed that atrophy of frontal cortex convolutions and dilation of ventricles occur, but the direct age relationship is variable. Computer tomography scans have shown a consistent increase of extracerebral space. Synaptic abnormalities (senile plaques), abnormal cytoplasmic tubules (neurofibrillary tangles) and granulovascular degeneration increase markedly from the sixth decade onwards. In particular, the last-mentioned is associated with the onset of dementia. There is also a deposit of a 'wear-and-tear' pigment known as lipofuscin, and a scarring which is associated with the loss of cells in some individuals. The functional significance of the yellowish lipofuscin is unclear, but it is said to be diminished *in vivo* during some drug treatments for confusion. Changes in axon terminals, presynaptic neuritis and decreased density of the dendritic spines have also been described. Densely staining intracytoplasmic inclusions (Lewy bodies) and neuronal inclusions occur in a minority of elderly people, mostly in those with Parkinsonism. There can be changes in the arachnoid and pia mater which become thickened and adhere around the surface of the brain and spinal cord. Even calcium deposits may occur in the meninges. The walls of the vessels are thickened and the perivascular spaces dilate.

Cerebral blood flow and oxygen consumption usually decrease with age. The method of xenon-133 clearance from the brain confirms this when the blood carbon dioxide tension is controlled (Fig. 1.3):

$$\text{mean cerebral blood flow} =$$
$$59.1 \ (0.34 \times \text{age}) \text{ml}/100\,\text{g}/\text{min}.$$

However, the arteriovenous blood sugar difference may be greater, indicating the greater extraction of oxygen per unit of blood.

It is disputed as to whether or not these changes can be explained by means of concomitant vascular disease, with more cerebral vascular resistance. In some dementias, with or

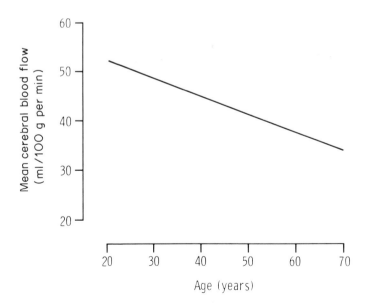

**Fig. 1.3** The relation of human mean cerebral blood flow to age.

without arteriosclerosis, reduced blood flow and oxygen consumption and increased vascular resistance do occur. Conversely, those with the highest mental test scores have better cerebral blood flow. The beneficial effect of hyperbaric oxygen in dementia is unconfirmed. The autoregulation of cerebral blood flow, under the influence of $Paco_2$ and blood pressure, does not appear to change with age. It is important in relation to spinal anaesthesia to recognise that in older patients there is less volume of cerebrospinal fluid, and it has a greater specific gravity.

A large number of older patients have some abnormality on neurological examination, such as absent tendon reflexes, loss of appreciation of position or vibration, or muscular wasting. Such common forms of stress as cold, trauma, infection, congestive cardiac failure or drugs may lead to confusion in older patients, and this may well be due to covert organic brain disease. It is important to remember that while three-quarters of dementias may be due to cerebral degeneration, the remainder are due to multiple causes, many of which are treatable, for example metabolic, toxic and vascular deficiencies or infections.

As one gets older, nerve reaction times and conduction times do increase, but the impaired sensory awareness of pain (which has been suggested as a factor of ageing) is unproven and, indeed, because of the indefinable nature of ageing and pain, may be unprovable. The size of motor units in the neuromuscular system diminishes with ageing as a result of the degeneration of some end-plates. Fatigue can develop rapidly, more units are needed for a given work-load, and there is a reduction of the maximum peak tension which can be produced. Underlying changes with reduced number and size of muscle fibres include a lower capillary-to-fibre ratio, thickening of tissue sheaths, and deposition of colloid interstitially. The electromyogram has typically less amplitude, and more polyphonic and prolonged action potentials.

## Electroencephalograph

The electroencephalograph (EEG) shifts to a slower frequency in senescence, the highest correlation being between the propagation of slow activity and lower cerebral oxygen uptake in those with psychiatric problems. There is a slowing (1 Hz per decade over 60 years) and decreased amplitude of alpha rhythm, with episodes of irregular rhythm in the theta and delta wavebands. Even amongst those not in hospital, careful analysis shows 50% of EEGs to be 'abnormal' in the old. The polymorphous EEGs may have prolonged latent periods for evoked responses: at first the slow activity is mainly in the frontal and temporal areas, and later spreads to the occiput. While continued fast activity in an older person is a good sign, slow activity over large areas of the cortex suggests severe mental change. The total amount of sleep diminishes little with age, but the relative percentage of rapid eye movement sleep is reduced, and there are many brief arousals and less deep sleep.

## Hearing

Presbycousis is a gradual sensory neural impairment which at first affects high-frequency sounds. One-third of the elderly population has a hearing loss greater than 15 decibels, but only a small number of these obtain aid for their deafness. It is common for the deaf to communicate by shouting because of the absence of auditory feedback and loss of voice power, and it requires sympathetic willingness to help the deaf when you talk to them. It should be understood that it is best to:

talk clearly and moderately loudly, without shouting,
talk face to face with good lighting on the mouth,
talk more slowly than normal,
allow intervals between sentences,
eliminate distractions, if possible,
make sure that any hearing aid is used correctly.

Because of auditory impairment, older patients have often learned not to listen to background environmental sounds, and they may experience a sense of unreality in a quiet room. Tinnitus, noise generated in the hearing system, and abnormal loudness perception can occur in the old, even without concurrent hearing loss. The prevalence of vestibular vertigo increases with age and there is a clear decline in the caloric nystagmus response (an indication of brainstem death) over 60 years of age. The eardrum of the elderly is less elastic, so that loculated middle-ear gas will be more rigidly contained.

## Eyesight

Nearly all elderly people have lost the power of focusing clearly on near objects. Glasses with increased strength of correction are necessary for close vision as the power of accommodation dwindles. With ageing, many people have a reduced capacity to adapt visually to darkness. Their pupils are smaller and the change of size with light levels is less. Both the size of visual field and the critical frequency of fusion of a flashing light are reduced. Some sensory isolation and disorientation may result as nights appear darker. Vitreous bodies (or 'floaters') are often present and bothersome. Everyone living long enough will develop cataracts after changes in the lenses of the eyes, for which there is no prevention. Glaucoma may be defined as intra-ocular tension greater than 20 mmHg. At the age of 60 the incidence of glaucoma is 3%, but fortunately this does not rise with greater age. However, macular degeneration is four times as common in the elderly and increases with each decade.

## Temperature regulation

The old, like infants, are less able to protect themselves against ambient temperature changes which are readily overcome by others. This impairment of regulation and adaptation lies in defective central control as well as in the peripheral effector mechanism. While the old may only discriminate temperatures 5°C apart, others can usually detect a difference of 0.5°C. Clinically it is best to use a rectal thermometer for central temperature monitoring as the mouth temperature is unreliable, especially as the old will not always keep their mouths closed. The standard clinical thermometer normally reads only above 35°C (95°F) so that a low-reading type should always be used, that is one reading down to 24°C (75°F). Accidental hypothermia does not require an accident, because

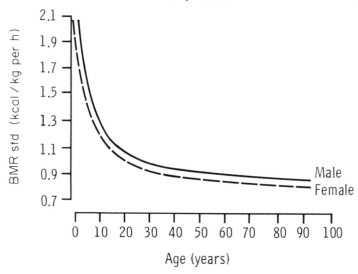

**Fig. 1.4** The relation of basal metabolic rate (BMR) to age in men and women.

the disturbance of thermoregulation occurs commonly with increasing age. Moderate cooling of affected subjects does not produce discomfort, and with a low resting temperature they do not shiver, raise their metabolism or vasoconstrict in the presence of an increased core-to-periphery temperature gradient. Even with normal thyroid function, the basal metabolic rate (BMR) is reduced with age, from 41 kcal/m$^2$ per hour at 20 years to 34 kcal/m$^2$ per hour at 70 (Fig. 1.4).* Diminished metabolism, due, for example, to myxoedema or inanition (and, of course, drugs), can contribute to producing this serious condition. Exposure to low temperatures at home and even in hospital is common and occurs even in mild weather. In a national survey of body temperature, 10% of elderly people in Britain were found to be at risk of developing hypothermia. Apart from the obvious dangers of hypothermia, such as arrhythmias, diminished cardiac output and impaired respiratory and mental functions, there are associated serious conditions which may lead to death. At any time an old, cold patient may develop ataxia, reduced urine output, pneumonia, stroke, cardiac infarction or pancreatitis.

*The SI unit for energy is the joule. 1 cal = 4.2 J.

Hyperthermia is less common but even more lethal. The aged, especially those with diabetes, arteriosclerosis, or Parkinsonism treated with anticholinesterase drugs, are prone to this danger when exposed to a hot environment (>38°C); sunshine is not necessary. The threshold to thermal stimulation is increased in both aged men and women, but to a greater extent in the latter. Impaired thermal regulation, due to diminished or absent sweating in the old, makes their environmental care crucial. The earliest signs of hyperthermia are apathy, weakness, fainting, headache, fever, tachycardia and dry skin.

## Cardiovascular system

Pathological processes increase so much with age that we have to accept those hearts with the least degree of abnormality as the 'normal' in the aged.

Myofibrils enlarge but are less numerous, while the calibre of the single capillary to each myofibril does not alter. Yellow-brown granules of lipofuscin appear at the poles of myofibre nuclei, accounting for the brown colour of ageing hearts. Brown atrophic hearts having a weight proportional to the body weight have long been described, but today's autopsies generally show a relative increase of average heart weight and left ventricular wall thickness with age. The atrial endocardium thickens and nodules grow on the closure lines of heart valves. Atrial muscle decreases as interstitial elastin, collagen and fat increase. The character of collagen changes (as in the lungs), so that the heart wall becomes stiffer. There may be amyloid deposits, especially under the endocardium of the left atrium. Increased density and sclerosis, even calcification of the collagen, produce loss of some of the bundles of His, especially of the left branch. Even distal bundle branches may degenerate and decrease. These changes in the conduction system make old patients very prone to arrhythmias. For some unknown reason, the number of pacemaker cells in the sinus node decreases with age. There is a progressive increase of coronary artery sclerosis with ageing. Vasomotor tone is decreased and vagal and carotid sinus influence may decrease.

The heart changes described above cause a limitation of

stroke volume, prolongation of isometric contraction and relaxation, with a decrease in the strength and force of ejection of blood.

### Cardiac output

Only cross-sectional studies exist and they indicate that resting cardiac output decreases 1% per year beyond the age of 20 years (Fig. 1.5). In sitting or standing subjects the drop with ageing is less. With exercise, at a given oxygen uptake, cardiac output is lower in the old. Because the old have lower maximum oxygen uptake, calculated maximum cardiac output with exercise is also lower. The reserve of cardiac output is limited, but the needful resting blood flow is well within the capacity of the old heart. If the reserve is exceeded, the early symptoms are fatigue, weakness, lightheadedness and focal neurological signs. The age degeneration of coronary arteries mentioned above is common, and occlusion with covert disease explains many cardiac anaesthetic problems in the elderly. The natural coronary blood flow age changes are slight, but maximum flow capacity is decreased 65% from that of youth. The resting heart rate is usually unchanged with age (cross-sectional and longitudinal studies), but the maximal heart rate has constantly been shown to be decreased with ageing:

$$\text{or} \quad \begin{array}{l} 210 - (0.65 \times \text{age in years}) \\ \text{approx. } 220 - \text{age in years} \end{array}$$

This could be due to a decline in sympathetic drive. The exact

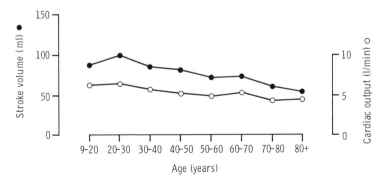

Fig. 1.5 The relation of stroke volume and cardiac output to age.

distribution of the lower cardiac output is not known, but all organs studied have shown regional increased resistance.

In general, total peripheral vascular resistance rises by 1% per year. The average flow of blood through the calf muscles is less in the old because vascular resistance is higher. Also blood vessel resilience diminishes as the elastic fibres straighten, split, fray and fragment. There may even be an increase in the quantity of calcium in the vessel walls. Collagen fibres stiffen and smooth muscle becomes thinner. The reduction of blood flow to the lips, the nose and the hands may produce cyanosis not related to decompensation.

The less distensible arteries and non-compliant vessels mean that a small increase in blood volume raises pressure sharply. There is a constant increase in the diameter and length of the major vessels, and this anatomical distortion may exlain the diminished blood pressure control, as baroreceptors in the aorta and carotid sinuses are damaged. Concurrent autonomic ganglion dysfunction is hard to exclude in the aetiology. The increase of heart rate and maintenance of blood pressure are less marked on tilting, and return to normality afterwards is sluggish.

### Blood pressure

The range of arterial pulse pressure increases with age. The difference in the diastolic blood pressure range is less than in the systolic, except in the obese. Cross-sectional and cohort data for blood pressure age changes differ, perhaps from differential mortality. Most population studies, except in primitive subjects, show increased blood pressure with age, and a majority of the elderly exceed 160/95 mmHg (the World Health Organisation hypertensive limits).

The blood pressure of cohorts actually ageing shows a rise of systolic pressure in both sexes, a slight drop in the diastolic pressure, and no change in the mean blood pressure. In women, the diastolic blood pressure is consistently lower than in men (Fig. 1.6). The adage that the systolic blood pressure is 100 mmHg + age in years is clearly wrong. These changes may be related to the fact that the elastic tissue in the wall of the aorta loses tensile strength while increasing in length and width (65y = 6.5 cm 75y = 7.5 cm diameter). Importantly in older patients, an increase of intrathoracic pressure, passively or

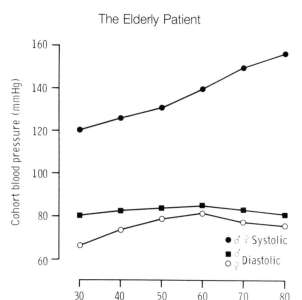

**Fig. 1.6** The relation of blood pressure to age.

actively, causes a greater decrease in blood pressure and little or no rebound elevation afterwards. Postural hypotension, whether spontaneous or due to drugs, is common in elderly patients and due to defective vasomotor control. Thus a fall in cardiac output or peripheral resistance may more easily precipitate syncope.

The total circulation time is said to be gradually increased with age: 48 s at 20 years, 58 s at 60 years, and 65 s at 70 years old. Arm–vein to arm–artery time is 19 s at 20 years and 29 s at 80 years. The important arm-to-brain (antecubital fossa to lips) values range from 15 to 20 s, with the average being greater with increasing age. Cardiac insufficiency may, of course, prolong circulation time, but infection, anaemia and hyperthyroidism all accelerate it.

## Electrocardiography and chest x-ray

The myocardial changes already described, and the presence of kyphosis and emphysema or other subclinical diseases, may explain the usual widening of the QRS (0.11 s) or increased PR interval (0.22 s) that commonly occurs with ageing. Notched T or QRS waves, ST-segment lengthening and flattening or decreased amplitude of all deflections are of little diagnostic value. There is commonly left axis deviation, therefore a right axis deviation of greater than 20 mm suggests hypertrophy of the left ventricular wall. Kyphosis and emphysema may hamper chest x-rays and therefore cardiothoracic ratio interpretation. If, however, the ratio is over 50%, it may signify clinical disease. Other evidence of importance in the x-ray will be the aorta's calcified and tortuous appearance when it is prominent on each side, with a knuckle, possibly calcified, at the ductus level (Fig. 1.7). Through aortic elongation, the innominate vein may well be pushed more cephalad in the neck. Systolic murmurs may occur in two-thirds of old people and are usually associated with aortic ejection or mitral tricuspid regurgitation. It is often very difficult to identify the murmur site.

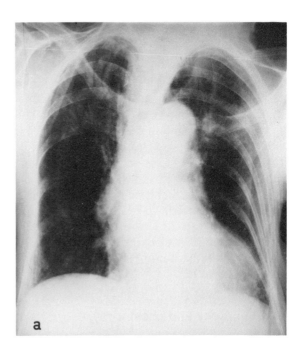

**Fig. 1.7(a)**  A chest x-ray of a patient in erect AP projection showing rotation of the patient to the left.

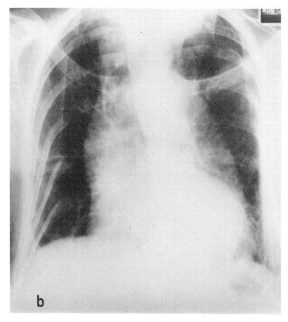

**Fig. 1.7(b)** The same patient as in (a) sitting. Film with poor lung expansion and, through rotation to the right, marked aortic unfolding which may be mistaken for an aneurysm.

## Blood

While 1 g% lower haemoglobin and a reduced haematocrit are frequent in the old, anaemia must not be assumed to be due to ageing. Old people tend to have low marrow iron stores, so that a small loss of blood may produce anaemia. Its treatment is usually effective and, if not, occult malignancy, chronic infection or poor nutrition should be suspected. A mild anaemia can be due to less available erythropoietin caused by a decrease of testosterone. Active haemopoietic marrow, is also replaced to some extent by fat, first in the long bones.

Old people normally have reduced immunulogical competence with thymic atrophy. Within the marrow there is a lymphocytosis and this is given as the reason for proneness to lymphocytic proliferative disorders and infections. There is also said to be an associated reduction of the number of T-cells. The mean corpuscular volume (MCV) is increased slightly, adenosine triphosphate (ATP) and 2,3 diphosphoglycerate (DPG) are reduced, and osmotic fragility and other minor differences occur in the red cells of old patients. For practical purposes, however, these red cells are indistinguishable from those of the young, and their life span is the same. White cells also show only minor subtle morphological differences in the old and the young. Relative leucopenia and lymphocytopenia are common, and the normal and high white cell counts are 3000 mm$^3$ and 8000 mm$^3$ respectively. Platelet morphology, counts and functions do not differ. There is conflict in the literature concerning clotting factors, and fibrinogen and fibrinolysis activity in the old. A higher erythrocyte sedimentation rate can be normal, but the presence of a normal plasma viscosity can be taken as an indication of the absence of infection. Plasma sodium, potassium, chloride, bicarbonate, magnesium and bilirubin levels are not markedly different. It is said that red cell potassium best reflects total body potassium. There may be minor changes in the total plasma protein, mainly due to reduced albumin, especially in ill patients. Alkaline reserve and the pH of blood decrease slightly, and more time is required to correct induced acid – base disequilibrium. Impaired protein synthesis due to severe illness can influence the T$_3$ uptake and calcium values. In the elderly, serum calcium (and alkaline phosphatase) levels have a greater range, even after correction for albumin variation. Higher ranges are also acceptable for serum cholesterol and uric acid, creatine and urea, and these may all be related to commonly occurring dehydration, regardless of renal function. The combined common occurrence of poor renal function and dehydration make the interpretation of the levels of many substances difficult. Free iodine levels are the same, thyroid-stimulating hormone (TSH) is higher and plasma iron lower, as is the total iron- binding capacity. Blood glucose is more commonly raised (? diabetic). Because of the frequency of atypical presentation of clinical signs it is convenient to utilise screening biochemistry in old patients. However, because of the overlap between results from healthy and diseased populations, it is important to decide the critical limit above which there is a chance of having a disease.

## Renal function

The renal nephron mass reaches its maximum at 20 years and begins to reduce at 60 of age. The reduction by 70 years old may be up to 30%. This is similar in degree to changes in the lean body mass and basal metabolism, both reflecting loss of functional tissue. From a plateau of one million glomeruli, atrophy may lead to one-half or one-third as many at 70 years old. The basement membrane of Bowman's capsule thickens, convoluted tubules hypertrophy ($\times$ 12), blood vessels of the kidney taper less, and the arcuate arterioles become tortuous with irregular lumens. It may be that this vascular change is the crucial feature. Compensatory growth is less, so that old donors are jeopardised and are best excluded.

All functional tests of the kidney show less activity with age. Glomerular filtration and renal blood flow are linearly reduced, the latter being thought to be a dynamic resistance phenomenon. In old age the glomerular filtration rate, renal blood flow and concentrating ability are half their levels in maturity (minus 1% per year from 30 to 80 years of age). Even the tubules are less responsive, and antidiuretic hormone (ADH) is unable to inhibit water diuresis as dramatically in old subjects. The maximum specific gravity and the osmolality obtainable are reduced. (The urine of the young has a specific gravity of 1.035–1.04 and an osmolality of 400, whereas that of the old has values of 1.022–1.026 and 280 respectively.) Response to pitressin decreases with age, but normal acid–base balance can

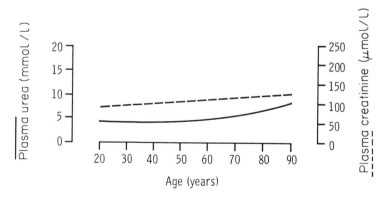

Fig. 1.8 The relation of plasma urea and plasma creatinine to age.

be obtained within a small range of adaptability. Large loads of acid or alkali can overwhelm the tardy mechanism. A blood urea greater than 8 mmol/l (48 mg/100 ml) may be normal (Fig. 1.8), but the renal reserve would then clearly be less and drug elimination could be affected. Whereas the serum creatinine is minimally changed with age due to a concomitant decrease of the muscular mass, there is a very clear-cut and marked decline of the creatinine clearance rate

$$\text{rate (ml/min)} = 133 - 0.64 \times \text{age (years)}$$

Water comprises about 60% of the body weight in young men, 52% in old men and young women, and 46% in old women. The total body water decreases together with the basal oxygen consumption (Fig. 1.9). Simple dehydration is a common disturbance seen in old patients and can lead to raised serum sodium and blood urea with a raised haematocrit and osmolality. The raised sodium has a blunt renal vasodilatation effect in old patients and conservation of sodium is also reduced. The total body sodium is less in the old than in the young (2500 mmol compared with 3000 mmol). As the sodium

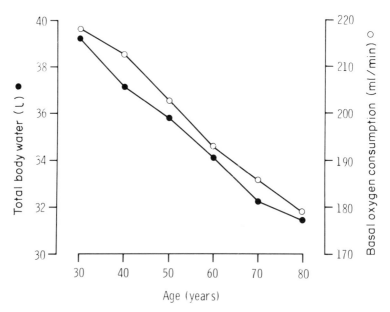

**Fig. 1.9** The relation of total body water and basal oxygen consumption to age.

in the serum is only 5% of the body store, supplementation for up to one week may be required to achieve balance. Sodium excess, on the other hand, is more rare and its signs (as with depletion) are quite indistinct, for example confusion, depression, apathy and weakness. Through poor intake and/or excessive losses, potassium depletion is common. Conversely, because of a less active renin–aldosterone system, aldosterone secretion is halved and there is a greater risk of hyperkalaemia in certain circumstances.

Imbalances of magnesium and calcium differ little from those of younger patients but are more frequent. For the anaesthetist, a most important factor is that homoeostatic failure after plasma loss is much more likely to lead to mortality in the aged. The chance of survival is slender, for instance, if the sum of the patient's age in years and the percentage of body surface affected by deep burns is greater than 80 (Boyd's index). Indeed, with any substantial fluid loss, shock may be insidious and difficult to treat, or, worse, it may not be treated vigourously enough because the patient is old.

## Metabolic balance

The changes in body constituents may explain the gradual decline in energy requirements from the age of 20. Up to that age there is a positive energy balance involved with growth. The subsequent small negative balance of energy is the essence of ageing, with diminished work capacity and reserve of organs and systems. The decrease in basal metabolism correlates well with exchangeable potassium or intracellular water and thus the functioning tissue. While water comprises less of the body weight, the change is principally a manifestation of a loss of intracellular water with ageing. The intracellular water also varies indirectly with the degree of obesity: body fat increases at a rate of 0.2%, albeit more in women and with a large range. The percentage of body weight as extracellular water is little changed (Fig. 1.10). Studies of longevity show some advantage for individuals with below average weight.

Absorption of glucose, fat, calcium, iron and vitamins are not as efficient as in the young. The rate of protein turnover decreases with age, and impaired glucose tolerance is common.

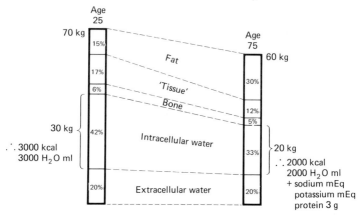

**Fig. 1.10** A representation of the make-up of the young and old human subject. The daily energy, fluid and some constituents required are indicated.

Although the energy requirement can be less in the old, the essential nutrients, vitamins and minerals must be provided in sufficient amounts. Multiple vitamin deficiency is common in the elderly and therefore their intake should be the same as in the young. Similarly, when any recommended caloric decrease is pursued, proteins, essential fatty acids and minerals need to be given in adequate amounts.

### Respiratory system

As age increases, the chest wall becomes less mobile and stiffer (decreased compliance). With dorsal kyphosis, due to degeneration of the thoracic spine and discs, forward curvature rotates the ribs and sternum forward causing a 'barrel chest'. The A–P to lateral dimensions ratio of 0.9 (instead of the normal 0.75) is often associated with the term senile emphysema, and this is contributed to by the less dense ribs which cause the lungs to appear more translucent. There is also reduced strength of the respiratory muscles and increased costal cartilage calcification. The elastic recoil of the lungs themselves is reduced. The main rigid constituent of connective tissue—collagen—does not increase but becomes aggregated and fibres bind so that lateral deformation is reduced. There is an increase in extensible elastin in the pleura and the septal tissue which, paradoxically, distorts the fibre distribution and hinders retractive function. A consequence of loss of recoil is that the lung volume increases and there is less efficient mixing of gas within the alveoli. The lung volume when transpleural pressure is at zero is larger in the old than in the young. Consequently its increase at other pressure differentials is also greater in the old. There is a small reduction of alveoli and internal surface area which perhaps explains the slight impairment of the diffusing capacity. Compliance of the chest wall decreases more than it increases in the lungs, so that the total compliance of the system decreases, but the airway resistance is little changed with age.

Both the inspiratory and expiratory reserve volumes, and therefore the vital capacity, decline with age (Fig. 1.11), but more slowly beyond the age of 65 years. The physiological deadspace–tidal volume ratio clearly increases and, less certainly, the functional residual capacity (FRC) is thought to increase. The anatomical deadspace enlarges because the diameters of both the larynx and trachea increase (127 ml in middle age and 155 ml in old age). A small part of the rise in anatomical deadspace is possibly due to an increase in the size of small alveolar ducts. A reduction of elastic fibres in the ducts

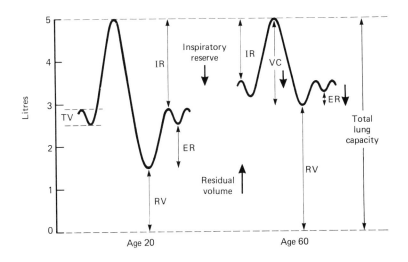

**Fig. 1.11** A representation of the spirographs of a young and old subject. The direction of change of some volumes with age is indicated.

and the mouths of the alveoli may explain why airway closure can occur in the old at a resting FRC. Any premature closure of airways must inevitably increase the residual volume. Unstable distribution of ventilation is very dependent on the tidal volume, which becomes more reliant on the diaphragm and abdominal muscles and is affected by a loss of recoil. While resting, tidal volume does not change with age, deadspace increases and alveolar ventilation decreases in line with the diminished oxygen requirement and metabolism. Alveolar – arterial oxygen difference is increased with a normal $Pa_{O_2}$ because the increasing inequality of the ventilation–perfusion ratio decreases the $Pa_{O_2}$. The accepted alveolar–arterial $D_{O_2}$ mmHg = 2.5 + 0.21 × age in years, or an increase on average of 0.3–0.4 mmHg/year with ageing. The $Pa_{O_2}$ fall is almost linear with advancing age, but the $Pa_{CO_2}$ is unaffected.

Normogram for expected arterial oxygen tension in relation to age (supine):

$$Pa_{O_2} \text{ mmHg} = 109 - 0.43 \times \text{age in years}$$
$$Pa_{O_2} \text{ kPa} = 14.5 - 0.057 \times \text{age in years}$$

Postoperatively:

$$Pa_{O_2} \text{ mmHg} = 94.3 - 0.455 \times \text{age in years}$$
$$Pa_{O_2} \text{ kPa} = 12.57 - 0.06 \times \text{age in years}$$

(see Fig. 1.12)

Changes in the pulmonary vessels include fibrous replacement of elastic media fibres and a reduction in the number of capillaries, so that there is increased resistance to increased blood flow. While the maximum oxygen uptake clearly decreases with age, this is related to circulatory dimensions more than to pulmonary ventilation function. Such uptake is decreased most in sedentary workers, therefore the muscle mass and its efficiency are closely related to the arterial lactic acid concentration.

Ventilation for oxygen consumption for a given work level tends to increase with age, which leads to dyspnoea without disease. The maximum breathing capacity diminishes (Fig. 1.13), mainly due to an inability to increase respiratory rate to as great an extent as when young. This is caused by a combination of chest wall rigidity, weak slow muscles, poor

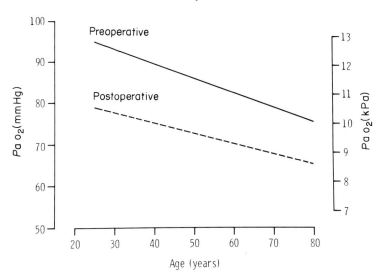

**Fig. 1.12** The relation of Pao$_2$ to age before and after operations (cumulative data).

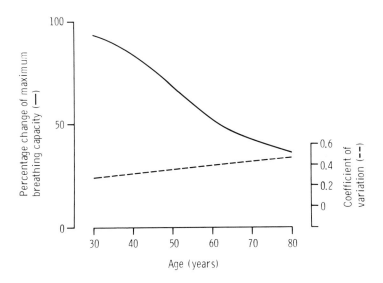

**Fig. 1.13** The relation of maximum breathing capacity to age, plus the coefficient of variation.

coordination and limited work capacity. Weakness of intercostal and accessory respiratory muscles makes coughing less forceful, and degeneration of the bronchi epithelium can lead to a less sensitive and efficient cleansing mechanism. With unresponsive glottic reflexes the scene is set for frequent lung pathology. Biochemical changes of the lung have been little studied. Whereas elastin increases, it does not correlate with amino acid changes, which in turn do not fit any structural or functional changes. Surface active substances have not been measured in the aged, which is regrettable as they contribute much to an understanding of lung mechanics.

## Gastrointestinal functions

The mouth of an old person is often dry as a result of poor fluid intake, mouth breathing, and less mucus from the glands of the palate. Gingival and alveolar degeneration and a marked increase in dental caries commonly lead to loose teeth, after a quiescence in middle life. Stiff jaw joints are not uncommon in the old. The state of the teeth, real or false, is related to meat consumption and haemoglobin level. Nutrition is also indirectly affected by reduction in the power of smell and the number of taste buds.

Varicosities of the sublingual mucosa vessels occur in half of those over 60 years of age. Cricopharyngeal and pharyngeal muscles are weak in a quarter of the elderly patients. Presbyoesophagus is a specific condition of the old in which there is delayed peristalsis and emptying, more from incoordinate than weak motor activity. Similarly, the stomach may empty more slowly and its acid secretion will be variable, with occasionally achlorhydria sometimes associated with mucosal atrophy, particularly in aged women. Fat absorption through the stomach may be reduced by diminished lipase excretion.

Animal studies suggest that there is reduced cell reproduction in the small bowel, which leads to shortening and broadening of the villi, together with a sluggish peristalsis. This may explain the common occurrence of malabsorption or maldigestion, such as lactose intolerance, in the old. In the large bowel there may be atrophy of the muscle and mucosa, an increase of connective tissue, hypertrophy of the muscularis mucosa, and atrophy of glands. These are commonly connected with the presence of diverticuli in older patients—half the women and a third of the men. Diverticular disease may cause extra motility, as will some drugs. Food acts as a cause of propulsion in the large bowel, but less so in those who are not physically active, and it must be noted that the range of frequency of bowel movement varies from three times a day to three times a week in 99% of people, young or old.

Most liver function tests show reduced hepatobiliary function with ageing, but not to a marked degree. In animals it is suggested that this is due to a related lowering of hepatic vein blood flow. Liver size is less and is directly related to body weight, but with some fibrosis and mitochondrial increase. Cirrhosis and fatty infiltration of the liver are not ageing phenomena, but liver damage due to toxic agents is more likely to be fatal in the aged. In old animals, drug-metabolising activity, especially oxidation–hydroxylation or demethylation, is less, but other changes in old people make such study results equivocal.

## Endocrine systems

There is a reduced adrenal response in the aged, which is clinically insignificant without exhaustive stress. Operative or postoperative exhaustion is not usually found, but through increased variability, the old may show a lack of response more often, especially those with malnutrition or depression. The sympathetico-adrenal function is well preserved in the elderly. In the old, the thyroid gland does not change in size; however, nodules are found in half the post mortems carried out and there is less functional activity with a reduction in the rate of thyroid hormone production. Thyroid gland physiology seems unimpaired but, as with BMR, the reduced activity is related to lesser lean body mass.

Simple ageing often leads to an abnormal glucose tolerance test, so that over 70 years of age, 25% of the population would conventionally be classified as diabetic. The reason for the impairment of glucose challenge is obscure; the insulin response to glucose is usually normal and prompt. It is unclear whether the delay (lag) in storage of glucose is physiological or pathological—it occurs in 11% of screened elderly subjects 3% of which are recognised without screening. For this reason, it is usual to use an upward revision of the glucose tolerance test. The limits of glucose abnormality with ageing rise 0.2 mmol/l (4 mg/100 ml) per decade. The fasting level rises 0.1 mmol/l (2 mg/100 ml) per decade, or the 'normal' post-challenge value of blood glucose concentration rises 0.5 mmol/l (10 mg/100 ml) per decade after the age of 40. Because of the likelihood of a raised renal threshold (elderly normal renal threshold 9 mmol/l (180 mg/100 ml)), glycosuria may not be present in a clinical diabetic. Endocrine upsets are described further in Chapter 8.

When considering the graphs of changed functions in this chapter, it must be realised that the coefficiency of variation is much increased with ageing, so that the older the subject, the more liable to error is any prediction (see Fig. 1.12).


## Pharmacology

The *coup de grace* for the frail old is often pharmacological and iatrogenic. There is a greater variability of biological efficiency in old patients, plus a common occurrence of disease. They have a decrease in active tissue and an increase in fat. Drug excretion is often decreased, as are depot distribution and metabolism. There is, therefore, likely to be more free drug in circulation. The target tissue distribution may rise and a heightened pharmacological effect will result. Absorption rate may be changed little; however, drug transport may be affected by a rise in gastric pH with a slower passage through stomach and bowel and a decrease in villi surface area. There seems to be little change in mucosal blood flow in normal old age, but diverticuli are common and may change intestinal flora. Because of the reduction of lean body mass and body water with old age, a drug dose equal to that prescribed for young patients may be excessive. The usual increase of body fat in the old will mean that drugs stored there will have prolonged action.

The protein-binding affinity of drugs may decrease in aged patients and plasma albumin levels will tend to fall. This affects both distribution and elimination for some drugs. Decreased capacity to eliminate drugs by kidney excretion or liver metabolism is the main reason for drug sensitivity in the elderly.

The glomerular filtration rate will control drug excretion in many cases (as with digitalis and aminoglycoside antibiotics), and hence there is a correlation between creatinine clearance and drug extraction.

Reduced tubular secretion causes higher blood levels of penicillin, procainamide, lithium and chlorpropamide. The action of drugs with a first-pass high extraction rate will be enhanced by the fall in hepatic blood flow. In old patients the presence of a sensitivity to barbiturates has long been known, and benzodiazepines have now been shown to affect the nervous system more, at equivalent plasma concentrations, than in the young. The concentration is liable to be less in those drugs which do not undergo oxidative metabolism before glucuronidation, for example oxazepam or lorazepam, but, as in infants, poor metabolism alone may explain the excess of side-effects in the old.

The possible reduction of the number or the pathology of receptors and the reduced homoeostasis which occurs with age, mean that more isoprenaline is needed to raise the heart rate and the propranolol blocking effect is reduced. The amount of phenylephrine required for a similar blood pressure rise is greater in the old, and greater still in hypertensive patients.

It is a common finding that elderly patients, especially women, have more adverse reactions to drugs. This can be related to the diminished reserve, so that the range between therapeutic and toxic doses is narrowed. There is also a common use of polypharmacy in the elderly, with an increased liability to drug interaction. Hypoxia, anaemia and hypothyroidism can make patients sensitive to narcotics, barbiturates and anaesthetics.

Drug interference with brain enzyme activity is greater in old animals. This is especially so with the drugs we so commonly use that excite or depress cerebral function, the disability being often worsened as sedatives or tranquillisers are pressed on those who are mentally disturbed. Any drug which interferes with catecholamine metabolism may cause extrapyramidal disorders. Compulsive restlessness, grimacing and parkinsonism (rarely oculogyric crises in old patients) are common with phenothiazines or butyrophenones. Anticholinergic side-effects of drugs, for example blurred vision, dry mouth, oesophageal reflux, tachycardia, urinary retention or constipation, are also more common and distressing with the elderly. It is best at all times to restrict prescribing to a small range of well-known drugs given in minimal doses over a short time.

Drugs that anaesthetists use, but which can cause problems are as follows:

1. Phenothiazines—produce extrapyramidal effects.
2. Benzodiazapines—cause drowsiness with confusion.
3. Opioids—produce dysphoria and sedation.
4. Hyoscine—excites and causes hallucinations.
5. Loop diuretics—cause low potassium in blood.
6. Digoxin—is often toxic.
7. Tricyclic antidepressants—produce hypotension and anti-cholinergic effects, causing confusion, urine retention and constipation.
8. Non-steroidal anti-inflammatory drugs—cause sodium retention and gastric irritation.
9. Sulphonylureas—produce hypoglycaemia at night.

Probably three-quarters of the digitalis given to the elderly is given unnecessarily, and it is rarely essential in patients with uneven rhythm. 'Classical' toxic features (nausea, vomiting, bradycardia) are uncommon, but increased heart failure, tachycardia, arrhythmias, mental changes (confusion and depression) and gynaecomastia must be sought as signs of overdose. Diuretics frequently lead to lowered serum potassium and associated apathy, malaise, urinary incontinence or retention, dehydration and hyponatraemia. Antihypertensives should only be given for those with marked blood pressure rise. Diabetes may be masked by thiazides, or exposed by perphenazine or steroids. Sedatives have been incriminated as a cause of depression, suicide, enzyme induction and habituation, or even osteomalacia. Antidepressants can produce giddy falls, glaucoma or urinary retention and, of course, the usual interactions are commonplace when polypharmacy is so rife. Older patients are receiving more and more cytotoxic drugs and any anaesthetics they require may interact with these drugs.

The following cytotoxic drugs and their interactions necessitate 24-hour withdrawal.

1. Cyclophosphamide with nitrous oxide, halothane or barbiturates causes hepatotoxicity and, by reduction of pseudocholinesterase, causes long suxamethonium apnoea.

2. Hydroxyurea with any CNS depressants or narcotic analgesics causes drowsiness.
3. Mitopodozide with halothane causes hypotension.
4. Bleomycin may increase pulmonary toxicity of oxygen.
5. Thiotepa may potentiate neuromuscular block.

In summary—with decreased cardiac output, renal blood flow, glomerular filtration rate, tubular function and some hepatic functions, the half-lives of many drugs are increased and their clearance decreased in the elderly. Since absorption is little affected, slow removal leads to consistently higher concentrations of most drugs in the blood. The picture may be complicated by changed binding to serum albumin or active sites, a decreased volume for distribution, and lower hepatic blood flow, affecting clearance of drugs with a high hepatic clearance. There may even be an imperfect mechanism of biotransformation, but much research is required into the effects of drugs given to older patients.

**Further reading**

*Biology*
Andrew W. (1971). *The Anatomy of Ageing in Man and Animals.* London: William Heinemann Medical Books.
Arnoll K.G. (1981). Cerebral blood flow in geriatrics—a review. *Age and Ageing*; **10**:5.
Becklake M.R. *et al.* (1965). Influence of age and sex on exercise cardiac output. *J. Appl. Physiol*; **20**:938.
Calloway N.O., Merrill R.S. (1965). The ageing adult liver. *J. Am. Geriatr. Soc*; **13**:594.
Campbell E.J., Lefrak S.S. (1978). How ageing affects the structure and function of the respiratory system. *Geriatrics*; **33**:68.
Collin K.J. *et al.* (1980). Functional changes in autonomic nervous responses with ageing. *Age and Ageing*; **9**:17.
Duke P.C. *et al.* (1976). The effect of age on baroreceptor reflex function in man. *Can. Anaesth. Soc. J*; **23**:111.
Edleman N.H. *et al.* (1968). Effects of respiratory pattern on age differences in ventilatory uniformity. *J. Appl. Physiol*; **24**:49.
Geokas M.C., Haverback B.J. (1969). The ageing gastrointestinal tract. *Am. J. Surg*; **117**:881.
Gerstenblith G. *et al.* (1976). Age changes in myocardial function and exercise response. *Prog. Cardiovasc. Dis*; **18**:1.
Gerstenblith G. *et al.* (1977). Echocardiaographic assessment of a normal adult ageing population. *Circulation*; **56**:273.
Haylick L. (1982). Biological aspects of human ageing. *Brit. J. Hosp. Med*; **27**:366.
Hodkinson H.M. (1973). Mental impairment in the elderly. *J. Roy. Coll. Physicians. (Lond)*; **7**:305.
James O.E.W. (1983). *Gastrointestinal and Liver Function in Old Age. Clinics of Gastroenterology.* London: W.B. Saunders.
Kenney R.A. (1982). *Physiology of Ageing—A Synopsis.* London: Year Book.
Kirkland J.L. *et al.* (1983). Patterns of urine flow and electrolyte excretion in healthy elderly people. *Brit. Med. J*; **287**:1665.
Kronenberg R.S., Drage C.W. (1973). Attenuation of ventilatory and heart rate responses to hypoxia and hypercapnia with ageing in normal man. *J. Clin. Invest*; **52**:1812.

Lange K., Boyd L.J. (1943). Objective methods to determine the speed of blood flow and their results. *Am. J. Med. Sci*; **206**:438.

Lakatta E.G. *et al.* (1974). Alterations in the cardiovascular system that occur in advanced age. *Fed. Proc*; **38**:157.

Leblanc P. *et al.* (1970). Effect of age and body position on airway closure in man. *J. Appl. Physiol*; **28**:448.

Lynn–Davies P. (1977). Influence of age on the respiratory system. *Geriatrics*; **32(8)**:57.

Malamed E. *et al.* (1980). Reduction in regional cerebral blood flow during normal ageing in man. *Stroke*; **11**:31.

McLachlan M. (1978). The ageing kidney. *Lancet*; **2**:143.

Port S. *et al.* (1980). Effect of age on the response of left ventricular ejection fraction to exercise. *New Eng. J. Med*; **303**:1133.

Raine J.M., Bishop J.M. (1963). A difference in oxygen tension and physiological dead space in normal man. *J. Appl. Physiol*; **18**:284.

Schmidt C.D. *et al.* (1973). Spirometric standards of healthy elderly men and women. *Am. Rev. Resp. Dis*; **107**:933.

Sestenbelith G. *et al.* (1977). Echocardiographic assessment of a normal adult ageing population. *Circulation*; **56**:273.

Shock N.W. (1961). Physiological aspects of ageing man. *Am. Rev. Physiol*; **23**:97.

Vargas E., Ley M. (1980). The assessment of autonomic function in the elderly. *Age and Ageing*; **9**:40.

Wahba W.M. (1983). Influence of ageing on lung function—clinical significance of changes from age 20. *Anesth. Analg*; **62**:764.

Wyper D.J. *et al.* (1976). Two minute slope inhalation technique of CBF measurement in man. *J. Neurosurg. Psych*; **39**:141.

Yamasachi T. *et al.* (1983). Correlations between regional cerebral blood flow and age-related brain atrophy. *J. Am. Geriatr. Soc*; **31**:412.

*Pharmacology*

Crooks J., Stevenson I.H. (1981). Drug response in the elderly—senility and plasma concentrations. *Age and Ageing*; **10**:73.

Crooks J. *et al.* (1976). Pharmacokinetics in the elderly. *Clin. Pharmacokinetics*; **1**:280.

Ramsay L.E., Tucker G.T. (1981). Clinical pharmacology—drugs and the elderly. *Brit. Med. J*; **282**:125.

Richey D.P., Bender A.D. (1979). Pharmacokinetic consequences of ageing. *Ann. Rev. Pharmacol. Tox*; **17**:49.

Triggs E., Mation R.L. (1975). Pharmacokinetics in the aged: A review. *J. Pharm. Biopharm*; **3**:387.

Vesta R.E. (1978). Drug use in the elderly: a review of problems and special considerations. *Drugs*; **16**:358.

# CHAPTER 2

# The aged patient

> I only began to live when I looked upon myself as dead.
>
> *J.J. Rousseau*

## Introduction

The grouping of aged patients into those between 75 and 90 years of age and those over 90 years (the 'longeval' in old terminology) corresponds to the division of infants into groups labelled neonate and premature. Paediatric and geriatric patients all require scrupulous attention to the details of their management, and the older or younger they are, the more vital is their need. In extreme old age the rate of senescence slows —that is, the regression slope in physiological functions flattens (see Fig 1.13 in Chapter 1). Patients aged 75–85 will, on average, live 5–10 years (Fig. 2.1), but in the case of the very old, they reach a point where continued biological existence becomes impossible. The expected human life spans, predicted from basal metabolic rate data, are 85 years for men and 98 years for women. At present nearly 3 million of the population of the United Kingdom are over 75 years of age, and it will be another 20 years before a reduced birth rate affects the increase in the number of aged. The ratio of old to young will be at its highest in about the year 2006, when 1 in 65 of the population will be 85 or over (Fig. 2.2).

The appearance of the very old is familiar but poorly observed. Loss of the outer third of the eyebrows is common, without myxoedema, and greying of axillary hair is a most reliable sign of ageing. Stature is diminutive—present centenarians rarely top 1.5 m (5 ft). The eyes sink due to fat loss, but the lips and abdominal fat deposits usually increase in size. At 85 years old the percentage of body weight that is fat is greater in women (45%) than in men (35%). However, this difference is larger at 25 years—woman (33%) and men (18%). By the age of 80, total body water (absolute and percentage of body weight), fat-free mass and cell mass all decrease by 7–14%.

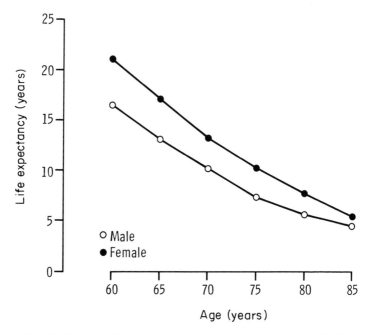

**Fig. 2.1** The average life expectancy for men and women at the age of 60 to 85 years old in Great Britain.

The ears elongate and appear pendulous, and the nails become hardened and mishapen. There is atrophy of muscle and replacement with fat, together with a reduction in the size of all organs except, perhaps, the prostate.

This general reduction of lean body mass, approximately to the proportions that obtain in the newborn state, is the culmination of constant change through maturation. Bones become porous and less substantial due to malacia, decalcification or degenerative change, and spontaneous fracture is a constant threat. Many aged people have flexed posture and they move with small steps using a wide base. Objective measurements of sway (Fig. 2.3) show a gradual increase with age until the patterns traced by recording devices are similar in the aged to those in preschool children. The old respond much less readily, with shivering and sweating, to cold or hot environments. They do not respond readily to thirst and thus fluid imbalance is common.

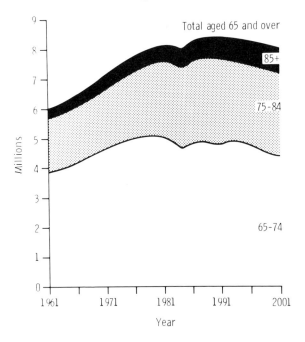

**Fig. 2.2** The recent and predicted number of people aged over 65 in the UK.

## Cerebral state

In the previous chapter the uncertain brain changes which occur with ageing were described. In the very old, the effects of cerebral disorders, general diseases and pre- and post-mortem changes confuse the picture. Decrease of brain weight becomes more rapid: the percentage of water increases at first, then the glia proliferate and the brain becomes surrounded by extracerebral spinal fluid in the vacated spaces. Octogenarians have a lighter brain than the young and a larger range of brain weights (in one study 818–2075 g). Those over 90 have an even lighter brain with more wasting, softening and cyst formation. The average nonagenarian will have a low cerebral blood flow rate (mean 40 ml/100 g per min, which is near the minimum for full neuronal function), less cerebral oxygen consumption and higher cerebrovascular resistance. The brain cells are special in that they are in a fixed postmitotic state and cannot, of course, divide; but it is far from clear whether a significant neural fall-

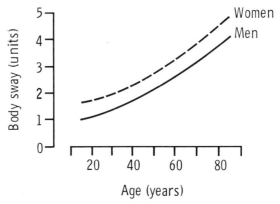

**Fig. 2.3** The amount of sway recorded in patients in units (one-third of a degree of angle) related to age.

out is a normal consequence of ageing, even in the very old. If the studies of mice are indicative, neural deficiency should only be significant in a few individuals after 71 years of age.

## Psychology

Old patients are frequently said to be confused when they no longer make sense of their social or physical circumstances. This condition has been compared with the occurrence of delirium in the young, but it is more common and easily provoked. However, the febrile convulsions and rigors of other ages rarely occur in the old. At one time, anaesthetists were taught the predisposing and precipitating factors associated with anaesthetic convulsions. Similarly, the predisposing factors, apart from advancing age, which precipitate confusion are pre-existing dementia, defective vision or hearing and parkinsonism. Apart from iatrogenic causes, confusion is most commonly due to pneumonia, cardiac failure, urinary tract infection, carcinomatosis or hypokalaemia.

It is usual to find that beyond the age of 70, 10% of patients score badly on any of the tests of mental state. These tests, particularly in their abbreviated form, are used widely, but data obtained from them may be misleading as repeated tests must be presented to each patient. The simple questions which are frequently utilised have been derived from earlier complex tests, for example an abbreviation of the Tooting Bec questionnaire (see Appendix D). They often include age, address, time in hours, location, recognition of doctor or nurse, date of birth (day and month), years of the World Wars, name of the monarch or president, counting backwards from 20 to 1, and repeating an address. When the very old have a low intellectual rating it can be related to a less labile cerebral blood flow, perhaps due to failing vasomotor tone.

Longitudinal detailed studies lead to the conclusion that intellectual deterioration is not correlated with age and, when decline occurs, it is usually related to illness or impending death. This is referred to as 'terminal drop'.

Psychologically it is as unhelpful to apply the epithet 'senile' to the aged as it is to apply 'puerile' to the adolescent. These are terms used for conditions which occur when there is a problem of communication and incomprehension due to unavoidable changes and stresses. Senescence causes marked functional changes which it is too easy to misinterpret with stereotype exaggeration. Enlightened medical schools now 'sensitise' students by having them experience mock incapacities of the type which the disabled old inevitably experience. Such helplessness can also be imposed by deprivation of stimulation and forced dependence.

Doctors have been known to diagnose senile dementia merely because an old patient had poor intelligence, not allowing for limited education or illiteracy. This partly explains the wide range of figures reported—severe dementia (or organic brain syndrome) in 1.0–9.1% of the aged, and mild dementia in 2.6–15.4%.

The life expectancy of severely demented patients is reduced by two-thirds, just as primary cerebral atrophy (Alzheimer's disease) and Down's syndrome seem to be associated with a genetically limited life duration. The term dementia is often misapplied, as it is a pathological medical condition which does not only occur in the aged.

A major change occurs in the cholinergic system; acetyl transferase activity, noradrenaline and 5-hydroxytryptophan levels are down, possibly due to loss of large nerve cells in the white brain matter and of trophic factors which stimulate compensatory dendritic branching. Physically, few people over the age of 85 can lead a totally independent life and it is quite regrettable that others may then decide on their quality of life, often with the best of intentions (see Chapter 12).

## Nervous system

In the old, changes in neurological signs which in the young would indicate disease, are frequently found. Thus the ability to discriminate smells, tastes and sounds diminishes, while the eyes accommodate poorly and the pupils react sluggishly to light. The small pupil of 'senile' miosis accompanies rapidly decreasing visual acuity for the majority. Examination of the fundi is obstructed in half the aged patients. Nerve conduction velocity decreases, on average by only 10% at the age of 75.

It is usual to claim that beyond 60 years of age the appreciation of pain becomes less obvious, but beyond 80 years of age pain thresholds lower, and there is evidence that older patients may complain less of pain. The interossei muscles waste to an extent that would be worrying in younger subjects, and many tendon jerks are less obvious. Abdominal reflexes are rarely obtainable. The speed of contraction of muscles, and of relaxation after contraction, is decreased. Extra muscle tone or tremor, especially of the hand and tongue, is common, while vibration is less clearly appreciated. The unique quasivolitional paratonic rigidity and clonus are more easily elicited but are usually of pathological origin. Thus neurological interpretation is never straightforward. Bladder and bowel sphincter control is less efficient in 10% of aged patients, but this is rarely permanent without a pathological cause. The volume of rectal distension needed to cause discomfort is markedly increased.

### Autonomic dysfunction

In the aged, structural random damage to the autonomic nervous system is related to decrement in physiological function. This is counteracted to a varied extent by increase in sensitivity of the system to neurotransmitters. The marked change in many aged patients' ability to produce a vasomotor response (Fig. 2.4) is crucial to anaesthetists. Impairment of the autonomic system in the aged has been associated with disorders of blood pressure control, thermoregulation and bowel or bladder function. A diminution of visceral pain appreciation has also been attributed to this. Other indications of dysfunction may be sweating abnormality, decreased lacrimation, pupillary abnormality and impotence. Many degenerative diseases to which the aged are prone, for example coronary disease, malignancy, rheumatism and bronchitis, may involve the autonomic system. Frequent involvement of the system occurs in neurological disease, for example parkinsonism or cerebrovascular lesion. Therefore some measurement of autonomic system activity should be used more often (see Chapter 4).

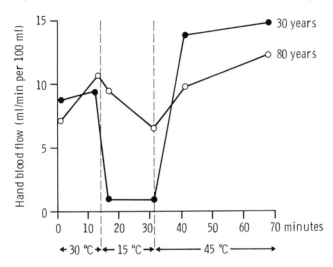

**Fig. 2.4** The hand blood flow changes in an old and young subject exposed to a period of cooling.

## Laboratory findings

It is usual to accept an abnormal as erythrocyte sedimentation rate (ESR) greater than 40 mm rather than the usual 20 mm. Whether normal ageing gives rise to a raised ESR in some patients is uncertain, so that it is of limited diagnostic value in the aged. In the aged, liver function tests can be normal despite a 40% reduction in organ size and blood supply. The gradual diminution of the basal metabolic rate throughout maturity usually plateaus beyond the age of 75. Vitamin $B_{12}$ and foliate levels, when reduced, must be viewed circumspectly as should patients with a haemoglobin level of less than 12 g

(15–18%) or lowered glucose intolerance (6% per decade decrement), as these are often temporary. There is a steady decline in the total body potassium, and a low serum potassium, due to low intake or excessive output. This may be associated with hypotonia or postural hypotension in some patients. In most of the aged the increase in blood levels of zinc, with a copper decrease in older men only, is not understood.

As the autonomic balance is less robust in a number of the aged, considerably less noradrenaline may be found, with a reversal of its ratio with adrenaline. Less cholinesterase (by 25%) and acetylcholine formation, plus a reduction in the number of choline receptors, will also affect the autonomic nervous system's function. In the very old patient (above 90 years), all clotting factors decrease and there are fewer platelets, but they adhere more easily. Neutrophils are more lobulated and they may appear to be less efficient. Immunological incapacity is likely to become more and more evident with ageing. A relationship between immunological incapacity and an increase in the frequency and extent of infective processes is most probable.

## Change in secretions

In men the gradual declining spermatogenesis and endocrine functions of the testes is common but not inevitable. This is related to the 80% incidence of benign prostatic hyperplasia in those reaching 80 years of age. The inexplicable increased conversion of androgens to oestrogens in ageing men may be connected with the high incidence of impotence. In women breast cancer is less liable to occur in the aged, while vulva, vagina, uterus and ovaries all atrophy to a varying extent. Parotid secretions have been found to be much reduced in the aged, and xerostomia from ascinar atrophy is also frequent. Achlorhydria increases in incidence in the elderly but usually decreases somewhat in the aged.

## Cardiorespiratory function

At 80 there may be a cardiovascular and respiratory function compatible with that which occurs at 50 years of age. The lungs of the majority of very old patients will have variable amounts of damage from minor infections, wear-and-tear, tobacco or pollution. The tobacco, smoked years ago had a very high tar content and pollution levels in urban areas were often very great. There is also a clear deterioration of lung tissue due to less blood supply and permeability and collagen changes which have progressed beyond the stage already described. It has, indeed, been suggested that the rate of decrease of $Pao_2$ increases over the age of 80 years. Nevertheless, the vital capacity and forced expiratory volume in 1 second do decrease more slowly over 75 years.

The electrocardiogram is likely to be 'abnormal' in half of the patients over 75 and all over 85, and over 30% of the 'healthy' aged have 'ischaemic' ST depression. Premature ectopic ventricular activity increases with age, and multiform, paired, bigeminy, or salvoes of such beats occur, but their significance is not clear (Table 2.1). Before an operation the electrocardiogram may pick up an unsuspected myocardial infarction or arrhythmia and is useful as a baseline for the interpretation of any postoperative recordings. In patients over 90 years of age, myocardial infarction (and indeed carcinoma) is less frequently found at post-mortem than it is in elderly patients below 90. The change in physical capacity with 25 years of ageing is like that produced by 3 weeks of enforced bed rest!

**Table 2.1**
*Abnormal electrocardiograms in the aged
(in order of incidence)*

| Abnormality | Percentage |
| --- | --- |
| T-wave changes | 19 |
| Q/QS patterns | 10 |
| Left ventricular hypertrophy | 7 |
| Auricular fibrillation | 2–5 |
| Bundle branch heart block | 5 |
| Ectopic beats >1 in 10 | 4 |
| Right ventricular hypertrophy | 1 |

## Polypharmacy

A third of all drugs prescribed are for the aged, so that three-quarters of these patients are taking a drug of some sort.

A third of the aged patients are taking four to six drugs at a time so adverse reactions or interactions are commonplace. In America the incidence of drug reactions is 1 in 4 after the age of 80 years. As in the elderly, drug therapy will be affected by changes which can be maximal in the aged. In essence, the delayed clearance from plasma and the decreased number of receptors which respond mean that most drugs act strongly and for longer.

The following are important pharmacokinetic changes which occur in the aged:

1. *Distribution changes:*
   a) Less body weight, therefore adult dose leads to greater mg/kg.
   b) Lower volume of body water leads to higher blood level of water-soluble drugs.
   c) More fat leads to lower blood level of lipid-soluble drugs.
   d) Lower plasma albumin leads to less protein binding of some drugs.
2. *Elimination changes:*
   a) Oxidative metabolism of some drugs is reduced.
   b) Liver first-pass metabolism may be less.
   c) Liver microsomal enzyme induction may be less.
   d) Glomerular filtration/tubular secretion decline causes slower renal clearance.

**Further reading**

Camm A.J. *et al.* (1980). The rhythm of the heart in active elderly subjects. *Am. Heart J*; **99**:598.
Foster C.S. *et al.* (1976). Sweat response in the aged. *Age and Ageing*; **5**:91.
Hamilton M. (1960). Rating scale for depression. *J. Neurol. Neuropsychiatr*; **23**:56.
Hanley T. (1974). Neuronal fallout of the ageing brain. *Age and Ageing*; **3**:133.
Howell T.H. (1981). Brain weight in octagenarians. *J. Am. Geriatr. Soc*; **29**:450.
McAlpine C.J. *et al.* (1981). Cerebral blood flow and intelligence ratings in persons over 90 years old. *Age and Ageing*; **10**: 247.
Novak L.P. (1972). Ageing total body potassium, fat free cell mass in males and females between 18–85 years. *J. Gerontology*; **27**:438.
Prakash C., Stein G. (1973). Neurological signs in the elderly. *Age and Ageing*; **2**:24.
Raftery E.B., Cashman P.M.M. (1976). Long term recording of the electrocardiogram in a normal population. *Postgrad. Med. J*; **52(7)**:32.
Titchner J.R. *et al.* (1958). Psychological reactions of the aged in surgery. *A.M.A. Arch. Neurol. Psych*; **79**:63.
Vahn R.L. *et al.* (1960). Brief objective measures for the determination of mental status in the aged. *Am. J. Psych*; **117**:326.

# CHAPTER 3

# Apparatus, monitoring and drugs

## Apparatus

There are many ingenious aids available for the use of old patients and those who care for them. Wherever these patients are treated, it should be ensured that helpful devices are obtained and used to encourage activity and rapid postoperative recovery.

Orthopaedic gallows (monkey poles), walking frames with wheels (for example Rolators), and high-backed winged chairs (Buxton or Chesterfield type) are indispensable in facilitating early postoperative mobility which is so important for elderly patients. Even simple ladder attachments to the bed foot and an extended arm device for picking up objects will be beneficial. Simple and effective hearing aids will help communication.

Extra consideration must be given when moving geriatric patients from bed to trolley and to operating table, because a poor transfer technique may start a necrotic lesion. This is because sores are caused not only by pressure effects, but also by shearing or friction which can tear subcutaneous venules and arterioles. A gentle lifting system, or carefully managed roller, should always be employed for moving the immobile patient (Fig. 3.1). Much attention is required to avoid pressure-point damage and nerve injury, so padding should be freely used, as should inflatable mattresses when required. In the ward, water beds, airloss beds or other such devices should be employed. Pump systems for intermittent compression of the legs, or electrical stimulation to avoid vein thrombosis should be available in the operating theatre and for postoperative use. All of these types of apparatus are used in the treatment of other patients, but it is clear that many have particular importance in the care of the elderly.

It may be helpful to have a full denture in place or an

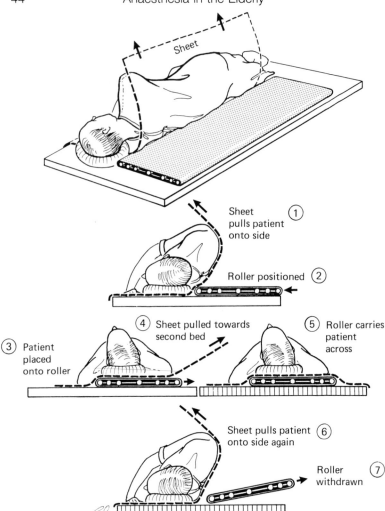

**Fig. 3.1** Illustration of the use of a transferring device which is helpful for patients and staff.

artificial gum shield when it is necessary to support the lips of a dentureless patient in order to maintain an airway. Very large facemasks which envelop the lower jaw and have inverted sealing edges (Everseal), may be helpful. Airways which are not as widely used in other patients, but may be effective in the elderly, are the latex nasal tubes and airways with an integral pharyngeal blocker (Beverley–Leach) or cuff (Brain). A fibreoptic tracheolaryngoscope is required for conscious intubation of the trachea when direct laryngoscopy is not feasible or permissible.

Accurate syringe drivers with a range of rate settings are useful for the administration of many drugs perioperatively. Self-inflating respiratory bags (Ambu type) are invaluable for the maintenance of ventilation during any transport of patients. Each transport trolley should be fitted with an oxygen supply and mobile monitors, for example a battery-powered ECG should be attachable. A 'third-hand' respirator on every anaesthetic machine is essential if other matters of care are to be dealt with without the physiological threat of apnoea.

## Monitoring

Appropriate pulsemeters, oesophageal stethoscopes, blood pressure apparatus and electrocardiographs are essential. Because ectopic heat beats are so prevalent, a simultaneous display of peripheral pulse wave and ECG is helpful because recognition of their synchronisation is important. Also, respiration monitors and metering devices should be freely used. Continuous display of the inspired oxygen concentration by an analyser is crucial with the elderly, who are so vulnerable to hypoxia during anaesthesia. A capnograph to measure anaesthetic circuit carbon dioxide is almost as essential but less readily available.

Nerve stimulators are essential for the proper monitoring of relaxants and they should be able to provide a train-of-4 stimuli. Central venous pressure measurements are more often required in older patients, and the necessary cannulae and transducers should be readily available. An over-use of central venous catheters is to be avoided because of possible serious complications. A soft, silastic polyurethane catheter is preferable to reduce trauma and thromboembolism. Routine arterial blood pressure measurement is essential because of the large sudden fluctuations which occur in stressed elderly patients. When a standard sphygmomanometer is inadequate an oscillometer, pulse detectors or Doppler device may be helpful. If continuous blood pressure monitoring is needed, plus frequent blood samples, intra-arterial direct cannulation of an artery is preferable. Data on age-related complications of arterial cannulation are not available, but extra care is essential. In some instances a cerebral function monitor can be helpful, but the routine use of EEG is not yet recommended owing to analysis and practical problems. Diathermy has to be applied with the recognition that in the presence of more fat, current requirements may change; DC defibrillators can be utilised without concern for age or size, but for the greatest success they should be kept close to where patients are most at risk of cardiac arrest.

Along with monitoring should go a strong sense of self-discipline, encouraged by enforcement if need be by a set of rules, within an anaesthetic department. Thus every anaesthetist should make a preliminary check of drugs and the anaesthetic machine at all times. There are unfortunately failings in some of the anaesthetic apparatus which has evolved. These can be overcome by the knowledgeable awareness of apparatus snares on the part of the anaesthetist and a high degree of suspicion of equipment failure in the event of a crisis.

For temperature balance, operating suite rooms should be able to have their heating varied rapidly. Microclimates must be controlled by proper covering (space blankets) and heating mattresses. Heat exchangers or humidifiers are needed in respiratory systems. Blood warmers are usually required for any but the slowest transfusion or infusion of other fluid. Patient core temperature measurement, from rectum or oesophagus, should be widely applied for major or long operations (Fig. 3.2).

The recent availability of expensive electronic devices to measure blood pressure non-invasively, electromyography, transcutaneous oxygen and carbon dioxide tension measurement, together with means of monitoring the anaesthetic circuit content, provides sophistication which is sorely needed. Cost and the risks in their use have so far limited the balloon-tipped catheter measurement of pulmonary artery pressure to a minority of patients in Britain.

## Anaesthetic drugs

The reaction of the aged to specific anaesthetics has been

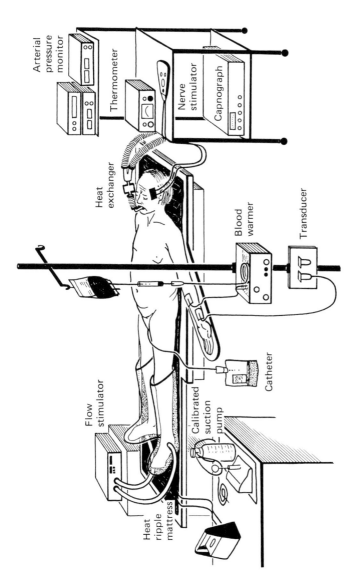

**Fig. 3.2** Some devices which should be freely used to aid perioperative care of the elderly.

little studied, but other pharmacological works lead one to expect a delayed, increased and prolonged response to most drugs. Any unwanted side-effects may be more profound and less efficiently counteracted by the body's protective mechanisms. The wide spectrum of effects of ageing and disease processes would indicate that some sensitivities are likely, but true differences in response to the drugs which anaesthetists commonly use are rare. Barbiturates and hyoscine can cause anxiety and restlessness and, as these conditions are very distressing to the old, such drugs are not usually given. Chloral hydrate or dichloralphenazone is safe, and popular hypnotics such as chlormethiazole are useful if their enhanced and prolonged action is recognised. Some benzodiazapenes are good premedication for the elderly—those drugs with inactive metabolites and rapid clearance such as temazapam and oxazepam. The routine use of intramuscular premedicants will be less predictable; they are poorly absorbed and the muscle depot is less available, but reduced protein binding may occur with the use of pethidine or morphine, for example. Morphine depresses respiration to the same degree as in a young patient, but may also severely derange respiratory rhythm (control). There is a probably slower clearance and longer duration of narcotic action.

The lengthened half-life of narcotics means that the one with the shortest, alfentanil, will be preferred as the old may eliminate it best. Fentanyl and alfentanil also have no active metabolites so will not be liable to accumulate. The active metabolites of morphine and pethidine will accumulate, especially with kidney dysfunction. Atropine produces less tachycardia in the elderly, but in small doses may cause more dysrhythmia. It has half the clearance rate and double the half-life in the old compared with young patients. An increase of intra-ocular pressure, which may rise to a dangerous level in those prone to glaucoma, can be aggravated by atropine or ketamine. These dangerous levels of intra-ocular pressure are, however, most dependent on hypoxia, hypercarbia or obicular muscle spasm. Neuroleptic drugs, while providing a stable cardiovascular state at operation, may cause postoperative depression and metabolic acidosis.

Irritant substances or irritating solvents are more liable to produce venous wall damage and consequent thrombosis in

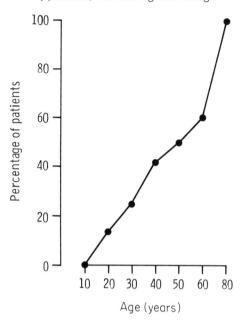

**Fig. 3.3** Percentage of patients of varying ages who have suffered from thrombosis after an intravenous diazepam injection.

older subjects, which is evident, for example, in the use of diazepam (Fig. 3.3).

The arm–brain circulation can be quite prolonged, and the potent intravenous drugs used may not have their maximum effect as quickly as anaesthetists are used to. Hence, overdose is a common occurrence. Such overdose effects may be compounded if the drug given is to be protein bound and a particularly old patient has a reduced plasma protein. This can be observed with the injudicious use of thiopentone, when any unbound drug may produce a deep level of narcosis and with it a profound cardiovascular depression. This can bring on a vicious circle of decreased binding to albumin and increased free drug with exaggerated action. Exaggerated dynamic action can lead to hypotension and reduced perfusion, decreased distribution and prolonged clinical effect and, possibly, cerebral hypoxia. Because there is less body water and cell mass into which the drug can be distributed in older patients, the blood level of thiopentone will be higher for longer than in young patients, and this will prolong recovery. The depression of cardiac output and heart rate caused by thiopentone is slower in onset and longer in duration than in younger patients, a difference which is not related to blood concentration. Thus the smallest amount possible should be used but, because of the individual variation, an exact induction dose is indefinable.

As inhalation agents have no similar pharmacokinetic disturbance they are often preferable, particularly as the airway is less irritable in older patients so that vapours are easy to administer. For the majority of inhalation agents tested to date, it is clear that the minimum alveolar concentration (MAC) value is reduced in the elderly: for halothane this has been found to be 0.64 in the 80 year old, compared with 0.76 in the average 40 year old (Fig. 3.4). Therefore the anaesthetic requirement for the aged is the lowest of all ages. The explanation for this is uncertain, but decreased cellular density in the central nervous system, decreased cerebral oxygen consumption or decreased cerebral blood flow have been incriminated. The increase in body fat of older patients means that lipid-soluble agents will accumulate and recovery will be prolonged to some extent. Also, of course, elimination of volatile agents by the lungs will be slowed by increased functional residual capacity and mismatch of ventilation and perfusion. There are few clearly defined differences in the use of halothane, enflurane or insoflurane in studies to date. The tendency of isoflurane to cause tachycardia is least obvious in older patients and their blood pressure may reduce less obviously. However, all the inhalation agents will produce further blood pressure drop with lower concentration. The biotransformation of enflurane to fluoride and oxalate may be nephrotoxic or lead to the formation of stones in susceptible patients, for example those with gout.

The intravenous and inhalation agents given, plus opiates, tubocurarine, phenothiazines and butyrophenones, may unduly depress the myocardium, and the peripheral vasodilation may be less efficiently combatted. Dysrhythmias and altered respiratory responses to anaesthetics are commonly described in the elderly, but are usually referable to existing disease. Hypothermia, for example, will clearly affect sensitivity to many drugs. While smaller doses are generally needed to induce and maintain anaesthesia, this is not always so, particularly in those with alcoholism or drug exposure.

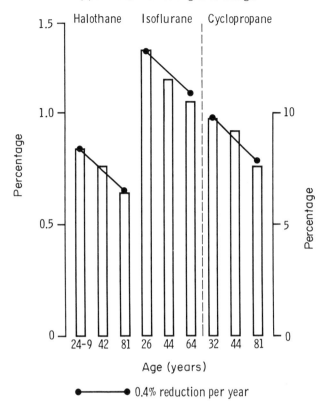

**Fig. 3.4** Histograms of minimum alveolar concentration (MAC) in per cent of agent for various average age groups. Each decade of ageing reduces MAC by only 4% of that of the youngest group.

Paralysis from myoneural block will be prolonged if there is a decreased tissue perfusion from any cause, as there is then slow removal from the site of action. There does not appear to be any clear sensitivity to relaxants with ageing, but the onset of their action is delayed, possibly through reduced cardiac output. It may take up to 6 minutes for the full effect to be apparent with electrical stimuli monitoring. Pancuronium has variation and a higher incidence of slow recovery in old patients, but tubocurarine recovery is less influenced by age. Altered plasma proteins correlate with the relaxant requirement, for example albumin and alcuronium, tubocurarine and gamma-globulin. Liver disease, malnutrition and debility may be accompanied by low plasma pseudocholinesterase and a tendency to long depolarising block and dual block. Hypothermia will also cause an increased potency of relaxants, whether by retardation of metabolism or excretion and less acetylcholine release, is not clear. Below 32°C the effects of relaxants may increase or reappear. Respiratory acidosis (with hypokalaemia) and metabolic alkalosis (with intracellular acidosis) enhance all non-depolarising drugs to a varying extent. For example, tubocurarine is markedly potentiated and alcuronium is little affected. Low serum potassium and sodium levels produce sensitivity to non- polarising relaxants, and high potassium levels lead to an anti- non-depolarising drug effect and an increased effect of depolarising drugs. The potassium released by depolarisation in the fit old subject is similar to that in the young—as is the plasma cholinesterase level. Chronic illnesses common in the elderly, for example, collagen disease, myocardial infarction, carcinoma, tuberculosis, can prolong suxamethonium action but this is rarely significant.

Relaxants are accentuated by low calcium and high magnesium blood levels. Enflurane and isoflurane are said to potentiate some non-depolarising relaxants, possibly by the reduction of reflexes. Relaxant and inhalation agent synergism may be valuable in old patients when experience with their control is perfected. Until then, much allowance must be made for the small muscle mass, and doses minimised accordingly. Atracurium and vercuronium have a more limited duration than other non-depolarising relaxants, and their action ends relatively rapidly. Therefore more monitoring is needed in their use and a continuous infusion may be employed. The two new relaxants have little cardiovascular effect. To reduce the cardiovascular effects of antidotes, edrophonium, which has rapid and short action, can be used because deep block to recovery is approximately 30 minutes. Because it degrades in plasma, atracurium is uniquely useful when a patient's liver and kidneys are compromised. Because renal dysfunction is common, gallamine may become a danger as it is excreted almost entirely through the kidney.

Free use of a nerve stimulator is clearly called for because of our limited ability to predict the effects of relaxants. This is shown by the following list of some drugs commonly used in the elderly which will interact with relaxants.

1. Cytotoxic drugs prolong suxamethonium.
2. Local anaesthetics potentiate non-depolarising drugs and prolong suxamethonium.
3. Quinidine potentiates non-depolarising drugs and prolongs suxamethonium.
4. Theophylline is an anti-non-depolarising drug.
5. Thiazide diuretics potentiate non-depolarising drugs.
6. Frusemide in low doses potentiates and in high dose antidotes non-depolarising drugs.
7. Beta-blockers—Phenytoin, diazepam, and phenothiazines—all enhance non-depolarising drugs.
8. Antibiotics—streptomycin, neomycin, polymyxin, cholemycin, kanemycin, gentamycin and lincomycin—all enhance curare-like drugs.
9. Lithium enhances non-depolarising drugs.
10. Chorpromazine, penicillamine, and corticosteroids may interfere with neuromuscular transmission.

Halothane 'hepatitis' and malignant hyperthermia are not as common in those over 60 years old, but their frequencies in relation to anaesthetic exposure of different age groups are greater and less, respectively. The dose of epidural local anaesthetic required for older patients is said to be less, but this is questionable. The number of segments blocked depends on the dose, and the level is higher in the old, but not linearly. The changes in membrane permeability can cause an alteration in the response to local anaesthetics generally. This permits success with lower concentrations which is also favourable because clearance and duration of local anaesthetics are longer in the old.

**Further reading**

Becker L.D. *et al.* (1976). Biphasic respiratory depression after fentanyl–droperidol or fentanyl alone used to supplement nitrous oxide anesthesia. *Anesthesiol*; **44**:291.
Brismar B. *et al.* (1977). The cardiovascular effect of neuroleptanaesthesia. *Acta Anaesthesiol. Scand*; **21**:100.
Chan K. *et al.* (1975). The effects of ageing on plasma pethidine concentrations. *Brit. J. Clin. Pharmacol*; **2**:297.
Chmielewski A.T. *et al.* (1978). Recovery from neuromuscular blockade; a comparison between old and young patients. *Anaesth.*; **33**:539.
Collier P. *et al.* (1982). Influence of age on pharmacokinetics of midazolam. *Brit. J. Clin. Pharmacol*; **13**:6021.
Dauchot P., Gravenstein J.S. (1971). Effect of atrophine on the electrocardiogram in different age groups. *Clin. Pharmacol. Ther*; **12**:274.

D'Hollander A.A. *et al.* (1983). Effect of age on the establishment of muscle paralysis induced in anaesthetised adult subject by ORG NC45. *Acta Anaesthesiol. Scand*; **27**:108.

Duvaldestin P. *et al.* (1982). Pharmocokenetics, pharmacodynamics and dose response relationships of pancuronium in control and elderly patients. *Anesthesiol*; **56**:36.

Falch D. *et al.* (1974). The influence of kidney formation, body size and age on plasma concentration and urinary excretion of diazepam. *Acta Med. Scand*; **194**:251.

Gregory G.A. *et al.* (1969). The relationship between age and halothane requirement in man. *Anesthesiol*; **30**:488.

Harrison G.A., Juniors F. (1972). The effect of circulation time on neuromuscular action of suxamethonium. *Anaesth. Int. Care*; **1**:33.

Havermark K.G., Wahlin A. (1974). Effect of enflurane (Ethrane) anaesthesia on geriatric patients. Preliminary report. *Acta Anaesthesiol. Belg*; **25(2)**:220–2.

Herman R. J. *et. al.* (1985). Effects of age in meperidine deposition. *Clin. Pharmacol. Ther*; **37**:19.

Hoffman W.E. *et al.* (1982). Cardiovascular and regional blood flow changes during halothane anesthesia in the aged rat. *Anesthesiol*; **56**:444.

Jung D. *et al.* (1982). Thiopental deposition as a function of age in female patients undergoing surgery. *Anesthesiol.* **56**:263.

Koblin D.D. *et al.* (1983). Age dependent alterations in nitrous oxide requirement of mice. *Anesthesiol*; **58**:428.

Linde H.W. *et al.* (1975). Cardiovascular effects of isoflurane and halothane during controlled ventilation in older patients. *Anesth. Analg*; **54**:701.

McLeod K. *et al.* (1979). Effects of ageing on the pharmocokinetics of pancuronium. *Brit. J. Anaesth*; **51**:435.

Marsh K.H.K. *et al.* (1980). Recovery from pancuronium: a comparison between old and young patients. *Anaesth*; **35**:1193.

Muson E.S. *et al.* (1984). Use of cyclopropane to test generality of anaesthetic requirement in the elderly. *Anesth. Analg*; **63**:998.

Schaer H. *et al.* (1984). Comparative clinical investigation of vecuronium, atracurium and pancuronium in elderly subjects. *Der Anaesthetist*; **33**:543.

Stephens I.D. *et al.* (1984). Pharmacokinetics of alcuronium in elderly patients undergoing total hip replacement or aortic reconstructive surgery. *Brit J. Anaesth*; **56**:465.

Stevens W.C. *et al.* (1975). MAC for isoflurane with and without nitrous oxide in patients of various age. *Anesthesiol.* **42**:197.

Vertanem R. *et al.* (1982). Pharmacokinetic studies on atropine with special reference to age. *Acta Anaesthesiol. Scand*; **26**:297.

# CHAPTER 4

# Assessment and preparation for anaesthesia

> Years, indeed, taken alone are a very fallacious mode of reckoning age; to the practised eye looks are much less deceptive.
>
> *J. Paget*

## Introduction

Any study of morbidity and mortality in anaesthesia shows that the young and the old are those most affected. Both groups have considerably less reserve in the face of stress than middle-life mature patients. In the older patients this vulnerability arises from the condition of the old (which has already been described) together with the increased likelihood of multiple pathology, overt and covert, and the many forms of treatment to which the patients are therefore subject.

## Routine preliminaries

We should be extremely careful in our preoperative assessment of patients and it should not be hurried or too limited. Time spent by the surgeon and the anaesthetist, with other physicians as required, in getting a patient in the best possible condition, makes anaesthesia and the postoperative recovery significantly more straightforward. In this preparation the understanding and motivation of the patient should be mobilised as far as possible, and this may entail repeated careful explanation. Whereas many older patients will acquiesce to treatment without demur, it is important to ensure that they are not fearful due to a lack of a comprehensible explanation. Care should be taken to reassure the patient who may be worried about the method of producing unconsciousness and the likelihood of waking or feeling pain during an operation.

A good history may not always be available, and a problem-orientated annotation may be helpful when there is multiple pathology. If it is feasible, an anaesthetic out-patient clinic for problem patients can be of assistance in the treatment of the elderly. This can ensure that necessary investigations are undertaken in time, certain preparations are properly completed, and a programme of progressive management is arranged.

A fine judgement is required concerning the length of the period of admission preoperatively. A sudden hurried, precipitate admission and operation may be as disturbing as a prolonged, seemingly inexplicable hospital stay before treatment. While day care and short stay are invaluable, one has to ensure that the social conditions and necessary nurse and general practitioner back-up are adequate. With the aged it is almost mandatory, for emotional and social reasons, to have perioperative admission of at least 24 hours, even for the most minor undertaking. Their associated pathology nearly always requires such an admission.

A listing of each patient's present drug intake is difficult to obtain and often inaccurate. Nevertheless, the history taken must include, as far as possible, a complete list of reactions and allergies and details of any previous anaesthetics which the patient has had. A recent chest x-ray (Fig. 4.1) and ECG, blood-urea nitrogen (BUN) or creatinine clearance and blood count, haemoglobin (sickle cell test in certain instances), together with any other indicated biochemical measurements are always required. If it is possible that the operation will be undertaken under local anaesthetic, this must be clearly explained and agreed to. It should be extremely rare for a trained anaesthetist to be unable to give a suitable form of anaesthesia for a necessary operation on an old patient, unless the patient is in the final stages of respiratory or cardiac demise.

Evaluation and preparation should be as fast and efficient as possible as the inactivity and isolation of old patients, which are almost inevitable in hospital, can result in their rapid physical and psychological upset—venous stasis, hypostatic pneumonia and mental regression, for example. On the other hand, if it is possible to convert an emergency into an elective condition through a more prolonged preoperative stay in hospital, mortality may be reduced four- to eightfold.

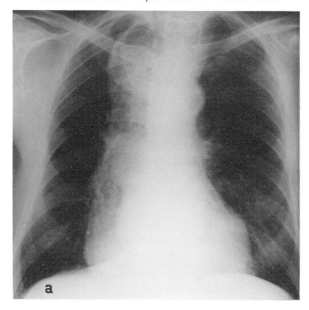

**Fig. 4.1(a)**  A PA chest x-ray showing widening of the mediastinum throughout the thorax. The appearances are those of an achalasia of the oesophagus with food debris within.

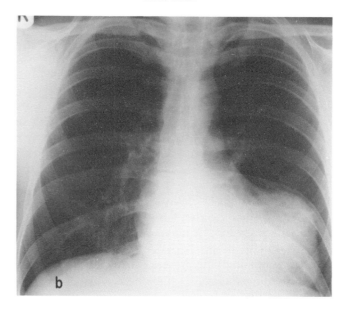

**Fig. 4.1(b)**  A PA chest x-ray showing heart enlargement. Configuration of the left heart border is highly suggestive of a ventricular aneurysm (confirmed later).

**Risk assessment**

Patients can be classified by their physical status. This is most commonly done using the American Society of Anesthesiologists (ASA) system which, while valuable in some respects, is not an indication of the operative risk and is liable to different interpretation by those scoring the patients. Anaesthetists have been shown to reduce the number of patients they place in Class 1 (with no disease) abruptly at age 50, while they sharply increase the number of patients who are a decade older in Class 2 and Class 3. The surgeon's and patient's view of this classification is more optimistic, especially in the seventh and eighth decades.

While postoperative mortality correlates well with the ASA rating, this merely indicates that the sicker the patient, the more likely she or he is to die. The system does not allow for the difficulties of the operation or the anaesthetic, nor for the age of the patient. More precise systems of risk examination indicate that many factors can be controlled so as to reduce the dangers (see Appendix E1). It is of interest that, in one large series of old patients given anaesthetics only 35% were rated as ASA Class 1. With the aged, life-threatening complications are so common that no assessment can predict outcome for individuals.

**Respiratory system**

When considering the respiratory system, the adequacy of the upper airway and its protective mechanism is important. The reserve of the lungs can be indicated by functional tests, but these are rarely helpful, except in the case of obstructive disease where the tests can be combined with the use of bronchodilators. The forced expiratory volume in 1 second ($FEV_1$) falls approximately 30 ml per year in men and 25 ml per year in women from the age of 25 (Fig. 4.2). The routine chest x-ray will show most restrictive lesions. The leakage of lung tissue which smoking creates can seemingly be alleviated by even a brief abstinence. If smoking is stopped for 48 hours, bronchorrhoea and carboxyhaemoglobinaemia will be helpfully reduced. If smoking is stopped for longer, an improvement

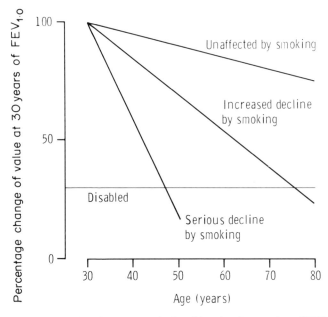

**Fig. 4.2** The relation of percentage reduction of forced expiratory volume (FEV$_1$) in smokers and non-smokers to age.

may be obtained in the cerebral circulation of elderly patients. Bronchitis and chronic obstructive airways disease, while of crucial importance, are less common with the passage of time, as there is less pollution now and the patients who were previously badly polluted have not survived. In the event of a patient having a cough, any sputum will cause a greatly increased risk, and culture and antibiotic sensitivity tests are indicated. Dyspnoea, which is less obvious in patients who are immobile and whose disablement has had a slow onset, is also critical. The importance of hyperinflation, or a barrel-shaped chest, is very questionable. What is imperative is that, when there is doubt, a blood-gas analysis should be undertaken.

Abdominal distension and ascites are clearly related to the alimentary system, but their end-result is often a severe impediment of the diaphragm movement, with consequent effects upon the lungs. The ascites, of course, also indicates the possibility of a severe lesion of the cardiovascular system or the liver, or carcinoma formation. Cor pulmonale is a condition which is too infrequently diagnosed; it is indicated by an increase in size of the right atrium or ventricle, with a pale peripheral lung and heavy hilar markings in the chest x-rays. Anaesthetists commonly state that poor gas distribution or a poor perfusion (that is, a mismatch within the lungs) is a major cause of hypoxia. While its aetiology is often imprecise, it is a pathophysiological condition which should be counteracted. It is a crucial part of routine respiratory preparation to educate the patient concerning the restriction of respiration after abdominal or thoracic operations and to emphasise the need to breathe deeply regularly and to cough frequently. Patients must be told clearly to overcome their natural reaction, which is to protect the wound and suppress deep breaths or coughs. Routine inhalation therapy, physiotherapy and antibiotics are called for in the patients at risk. The commonest risk factors for pulmonary complications are left ventricular heart failure, pre-existing pulmonary disease, reduced peak flow rates and long or repeated operations on the trunk.

## Cardiovascular system

Incipient heart failure may be suggested by a feeling of suffocation at night or a persistent cough. A past history of oedema of the legs, dyspnoea and foaming of sputum is most important as an indication of previous decompensation. Any angina pectoris is important, particularly when it is recent and increasing in severity. The usual signs of heart failure, such as pallor, cyanosis, neck vein distension and pulsation, pulmonary congestion, hepatomegalia, ascites, peripheral oedema or, in the case of those who have been supine for any length of time, presacral oedema, must never be considered as normal signs of ageing.

Since non-specific ST segment and T-wave changes in the ECG are common in the aged, they are not of great clinical importance preoperatively. The ECG, nevertheless, is invaluable as a baseline and, in the case of heart block, the type of block will indicate whether preoperative pacing is essential. Anaesthesia may cause arrhythmias, premature beats, or reduced atrio-ventricular (A-V) conduction, and it may change cardiac excitability itself, or in combination with blood transfusion or overventilation. Thus, a temporary pacemaker insertion may be needed for an operation alone. This is mandatory where there is a history of Stokes–Adams attacks, or unexplained blackouts with ECG evidence of an AV or bifascicular block. Severe bradycardia (with or without auricular fibrillation) accompanied by cardiac failure, angina or fainting, also indicates a need for temporary pacing.

Even without symptoms, a third-degree or incomplete AV block (Mobitz type 2 block) requires insertion of a temporary pacemaker. With the pacemaker *in situ* it is important to be aware of factors affecting the conduction threshold. With an increased threshold, pacing may fail, and with a decreased threshold ventricular fibrillation may ensue. Suxamethonium, hyperkalaemia or acid–base imbalance may increase the conduction threshold. A decrease of the conduction threshold involves myocardial ischaemia due to cardiac output fall, bleeding, high intermittent positive-pressure ventilation (IPPV) or drug overdose.

When pacemakers first became available, patients presenting for operations with a heart block were, in some institutions, routinely provided with a standby cardiac pacemaker preoperatively. It is now known that there are certain hazards involved with pacemaker application, and that in prospective studies of patients with first-degree or partial bundle branch block, even with left axis deviation and possibly right axis deviation, there is no need for a pacemaker insertion. This may also apply in the case of a PR interval prolongation, although specialist advice may be helpful with such patients. All these patients, of course, must be monitored throughout the procedure with an electrocardiograph.

The importance of an asymptomatic heart murmur is decided by clinical examination. Very loud murmurs which are detected at the back of the chest and have a palpable thrill, can be assumed to be of organic origin. Innocent murmurs—that is, those which are not organic—are often said to be quieter and more superficial, varying with respiration and distinctly localised to the left of the sternum.

The symptoms and presentation of myocardial infarction in the aged must be clearly understood. The classical symptom of a prolonged bout of pain only afflicts the minority of cases. The atypical presentations are confusion, dyspnoea, hypotension, infarction from arterial embolism elsewhere in the body, vomiting and weakness. Some cases are completely silent and only discovered with the ECG. Any ECG deviation must be viewed in the light of clinical signs and symptoms, because transient arrhythmias are much more common in old patients, but these can be relatively benign and not correlated with future heart problems (see Table 2.1 in Chapter 2).

In some centres, the product of heart rate and systolic blood pressure is utilised as a measure of the coronary circulation. Products between 12 000 and 20 000 are arbitrarily recommended. Assessment of the resting, tolerated 'exercise' and anginal rates for each patient may be helpful. Increased heart rate may produce more ischaemia than hypertension, so that keeping the rate below 90 beats/min is recommended for those at risk.

In a large study of patients undergoing anaesthesia and surgery the overall reinfarction rate within 1 week of patients who had had a previous infarction was approximately 6%, of which over half died. More importantly, the incidence of reinfarction was much greater the closer it was to the first infarction —under 3 months 27%, under 6 months 11%, and over 6 months 5%—so operations should be postponed whenever possible in these patients, particularly if they require major chest or abdominal work, if the anaesthetic and operation may be prolonged, or if they suffer from hypertension. Neither the type of previous infarction nor the presence of angina or diabetes creates extra risk. The age of the patient is not significantly related to an increased risk either. Thus the common risk factors for cardiac complications are myocardial infarction, unstable angina and pulmonary congestion.

*Deep vein thrombosis*

Any elderly patient who is to undergo a major operation is a potential victim of deep vein thrombosis and pulmonary embolism. Obesity, cardiovascular disease, varicose veins or a history of deep vein thrombosis or pulmonary embolism, as well as some blood dyscrasias and immunosuppressive therapy, produce an increased risk and call for preventive measures, especially in certain operations. As there are a variety of methods advocated to prevent deep vein thrombosis, it is helpful to calculate the expected incidence of this condition postoperatively.

In the old with extensive operations, there is an increase in malignant disease, inflammatory disease and postoperative infection, or any condition that reduces the mobility of the patient. For those with a history of recent venous thrombo-embolism, pelvic–abdominal, prostate or hip surgery, and no prophylaxis, the incidence of peripheral venous thrombosis is up to 60%, and 20% may have proximal vein thrombosis, with 1–2% succumbing to pulmonary embolism.

Compression stockings, intermittent pneumatic compression, anticoagulants and dextran 70 infusion all appear to have some prophylactic effect if they are used operatively and continued during the period of immobilisation. Because of the ease of administration the 8-hourly low-dose heparin regime is widely applied (5000 units administered subcutaneously 2 hours preoperatively and continued postoperatively). This will halve the incidence of thrombosis and embolism but is associated with a risk of bleeding, particularly when administered to the elderly for more than 48 hours. In one study a combination of heparin and dextran increased the incidence of pulmonary embolism, but the use of coumarin and dextran 70 was effective. Oral anticoagulants can be used, but the maintenance of the correct degree of control value is difficult. If an infusion pump is used for heparin, it is adjusted to maintain heparin levels of approximately 0.1 ng/ml (1.25–1.5 times the control partial thromboplastin time, PPT). A continuous administration of a *very* low dose (1 I.U./kg/h) of heparin may be effective with minimal risk of haemorrhage.

Preoperative prophylactic digitalisation of aged patients is not advisable. The prevention of irregularities caused by anaesthesia or surgery by the use of digitalis is, even in patients with heart disease, uncertain and must be balanced against the risk of digitalis-induced arrhythmias, especially in view of the frequency of hypokalaemia and alkalosis amongst the elderly. Digitalisation is best limited to patients in heart failure, with fast atrial fibrillation or with frequent premature beats. Discretionary use of digitalis may be made for patients having major abdominal or chest operations after myocardial infarction or ventricular disorders. Digitalisation in geriatric anaesthesia should be seen in the light of its narrow therapeutic concentration (for digoxin 1–2 ng/ml), the overlap of therapeutic and toxic concentrations (3 ng/ml) and the heightened sensitivity of the old due to their having less muscle for the drug to be bound to. Any cardiotoxicity requires operative delay, if possible, and treatment. Rapid digitalisation is problem prone, and when used to increase cardiac output it should be as controlled as dopamine or isoprenaline infusions. It is in patients with questionable cardiac output that sophisticated forms of monitoring, such as central venous pressure, pulmonary artery pressure and intra-arterial pressure, may be indicated. The placement of a pulmonary artery catheter for monitoring is particularly contentious. It is a difficult procedure, not innocuous, but expensive, yet in patients over 65 years old 9 out of 10 so monitored would be considered to have cardiac dysfunction.

Central venous pressure measurement is an expression of the balance between right atrial filling and cardiac output. In the presence of shock, a level of 5 cm $H_2O$ indicates low blood volume, while a failing heart is revealed by 15-cm levels. Even in old patients, pulmonary oedema is rare with a central venous pressure (CVP) measurement of 15 cm $H_2O$ or less.

### Hypertension

Arteriosclerosis and hypertension are common in the aged, and their importance for the anaesthetist resides in the fact that the heart in such patients will not be normal; the brain and the kidneys are also liable to have a serious reduction of their reserves. If the patient's hypertension is controlled by drugs, the consensus view is that they should continue to be administered, even at the risk of some interactions. For the uncontrolled, markedly hypertensive patient, it is wise to have admission with bed rest and continuous blood pressure recording, and the indicated antihypertensive drugs should be effective before the operation. Untreated hypertensive patients can suffer marked hypotension with anaesthesia —conduction spinal block being especially hazardous.

Beta-receptor blocking drugs are frequently used for hypertension, heart ischaemia, cardiomyopathies and dysrhythmia. As dysrhythmias, high blood pressure and even ischaemia with cardiac arrest may occur when these drugs are discontinued, it is now recommended that adrenergic blockage is maintained. Responses during induction and maintenance of anaesthesia are important and dependent on the agents and methods used. The interaction of ether and cyclopropane may be more adverse than that of newer anaesthetics, but reflex responses are more method dependent (see Chapter 5).

Most other antihypertensive drugs (apart from diuretics) act by dilating arterioles, and their interaction with anaesthetic drugs is not as important as the presence of ischaemia of the heart or cerebrovascular disease. Withdrawal of these drugs may lead to a hypertensive crisis, whereas maintenance of treatment provides a more stable patient.

One group of drugs most commonly prescribed for the elderly is diuretics, with or without potassium supplant. For any patient who is on, or likely to be on, a diuretic form of treatment, the serum potassium level should be estimated within 24 hours of the operation. With congestion of the lungs or peripheral tissues, diuretics may be the most valuable treatment, as long as serum electrolytes are carefully monitored.

## Renal system

The aged patient's renal function is usually adequate for normal living. However, when severe metabolic changes occur because of the diminished tubular reabsorption, excretion and concentration ability, the volume of urine necessary to handle the solutes has to be increased. It must be stressed that, with retention of sodium, there must be sparing administration, particularly when a quarter of the total body sodium is not exchangeable. Of the total potassium content of the body, however, only 0.05% is not exchangeable. The average diet contains 100 mmol (mEq) of salt per day, but there is only about half that amount of potassium. Because the kidneys do not conserve potassium, a large deficit can occur within a few days if intake is inadequate. Clinical evaluation of the kidneys is dependent on weight changes and measurement and analysis of body fluids, including urine.

### Fluid and electrolytes

In general, the latitude for improper fluid and electrolyte therapy is not as great in dealing with elderly patients. Fluid intake should be approximately 1500–2000 ml per day. If extensive surgery is performed, the maximal response to stress is elicited and further curtailment of fluid may be necessary. When there is loss of fluids due to drainage, fistuli, diarrhoea or vomiting, it is, of course, necessary to replace them volume for volume. In the case of lower intestinal secretions, normal saline is used, whereas half-normal saline is used for gastric secretions.

The potassium need is less urgent with surgery, without diuretics having been used, and it is usual to limit the amount to 40 mmol/l (mEq/l) per day in the first instance. There must be adequate urine output before potassium is administered. The carbohydrate need for the elderly is not clear, but 50 g daily (1 litre of 5% dextrose) is the smallest amount which will diminish protein breakdown and further potassium loss or kidney overwork.

Metabolic acidosis is a common occurrence with kidney dysfunction. Acidaemia is associated with a raised, and alkalaemia and a lowered serum potassium (approximately 0.5 mmol (mEq) of potassium per 0.1 pH unit change). There is a crucial connection between respiratory alkalosis and a low serum potassium: in such instances the potassium is driven into the cells and creates a great potassium need. This is important when metabolic acidosis follows hypoventilation, when the amount of potassium may be crucial to heart function. Metabolic alkalosis is a rare consequence of excessive vomiting and is apparently not as dangerous. The measurement of blood urea and creatinine clearance is essential to indicate kidney function, and, if the blood chemistry is in disarray, dialysis may be necessary before any operation.

As in the care of neonates, the anaesthetist must be constantly aware of the possibility of water depletion in old patients. Signs of this may be unimpressive until it is quite severe. The skin becomes dry and lacks turgor (juiciness), the tongue is dry and furred, and the patient is often lethargic. It may be necessary to obtain the electrolyte values from venous blood, which will indicate the diagnosis by their increased concentration for example serum sodium >155 mmol/l (mEq/l) and potassium >5 mmol/l (mEq/l). The urine flow will be low and the urine highly coloured, with an increase of specific gravity, while the blood urea level is often raised. The amount of fluid needed for replacement can be roughly gauged by the formula:

$$\text{Volume (litres)} = \frac{\text{serum sodium mmol/l (mEq/l)} - 140 \times \text{body weight (kg)}}{200}$$

If, conversely, there is a low serum sodium level (<132 mmol/l, mEq/l), this can be caused by any of a number of conditions which are also found in young patients. In extreme cases there will be associated water intoxication and acid–base disturbance, together with potassium depletion, so pH, $Paco_2$, serum potassium and bicarbonate levels must be measured. Clinical signs of the extreme form of this condition are sunken eyes, low eyeball tension, and a dry upper airway which makes speech and swallowing difficult. Afflicted patients have a gaunt, desiccated appearance and the folds of their skin remain deformed when pinched. Finally, they suffer a reduction in jugular vein pressure, cardiac output, peripheral pulse and blood pressure, and such a gross loss of blood volume that severe shock may be apparent. The major causes of low serum sodium levels are the loss of upper intestinal secretions, severe water diarrhoea and renal loss of sodium.

Other forms of hyponatraemia are associated with heart failure, iatrogenic causes, excessive ADH effect and the sick cell syndrome, all of which require expert medical advice. Confirmatory ECG signs of abnormal potassium levels are important as they are a warning of the arrhytmias that may occur (Fig. 4.3). Prolonged use of a loop diuretic, or even a short intensive course, may produce hypokalaemia or hypomagnaemia very readily in the elderly. With a low serum magnesium, when intracellular levels may be lower, the symptoms of depression, muscle weakness and artrial fibrillation, refactory to digoxin, can occur. If the level is less than 0.7 mmol/l (1.7 mg/100 ml), magnesium sulphate 10 mmol/day should be administered. Apart from diuretic treatment, local soft water, poor dietary intake and alcoholism predispose patients to this condition.

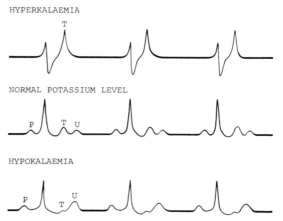

**Fig. 4.3** A Diagram of the classical electrocardiogram with differing levels of plasma potassium.

## Steroid supplementation

Any patient on steroid therapy may be considered for extra cortisone treatment during or after an operation for any endogenous deficiency of that stress hormone. Also patients who have been treated with steroids within 2 months of an operation may well suffer from suppression of their own adrenal cortex and will therefore require fortification before they can be anaesthetised. One school of opinion maintains no extra steroid is required for minor operations, provided there is careful observation postoperatively. For intermediate operations, one single dose of soluble hydrocortisone hemisuccinate may be sufficient, if there is careful, continuous observation. For major operations, the usual regimen is a 100-mg hydrocortisone intramuscular injection every 6 hours from the premedication to 2–3 days later. Some anaesthetists stop the parenteral steroid suddenly, while others prefer a gradual reduction. The advocates of these varying regimens all advise hydrocortisone treatment for any unexplained hypotension. As complications with hydrocortisone are very rare, the older patient is so vulnerable and monitoring so variable, it is the author's opinion that a regular regimen of cover is advisable, except in the most minor operation when patients have had very small amounts of steroid preoperatively.

## Diabetes

Many older diabetic patients have a mild form of the disease, but a neuropathy may exist which can be of great importance as it can cause respiratory arrest perioperatively. Also gastroparesis, with consequent delay in stomach emptying may be of importance with anaesthetic management. Some of the oral antidiabetic drugs have a prolonged effect and may require withdrawal over 2 or 3 days. Owing to the common elevation of the renal glucose threshold in the elderly, a random blood sugar screening test is indicated. The common, mild diabetes of the elderly (see Chapter 7) is frequently managed by diet, or diet and oral drugs together. The disease may get out of control, due to the condition for which the operation is required, or due to the stress of the operation itself, so blood sugar must be determined perioperatively.

If the patient is on oral hypoglycaemic drugs and has a preoperative blood sugar greater than 11 mmol/1 (200 mg/100 ml) then insulin administration is required pre- and postoperatively until feeding is resumed. Of special concern is the most commonly used sulphonylurea drug chlorpropamide, as it must be withdrawn for 24 hours before fasting, and a glucose infusion may be needed to avoid hypoglycaemia; this is because chlorpropamide's half-life is about 36 hours. It must be remembered that the hypoglycaemia that may occur can be aggravated if the patient is on coumarin or beta-blocking agents. The patients who are being treated with delayed action insulin are subject to the same problem, as the drug may also last 16–36 hours. For the perioperative period, quick-acting soluble insulin is preferred because there is a constant change of need which must be monitored by blood sugar assay.

There is no great danger of hypoglycaemia with maturity-onset diabetic patients, so a saline infusion may be suitable. If an energy supply is thought to be necessary to avoid fatty acid utilisation and consequent ketoacidosis, 1 litre of 5% glucose (50 g) can be administered with blood sugar measurements every 8 hours. Although modern anaesthesia and surgery precipitate a lower blood sugar rise, it must not be forgotten that an increase of insulin requirement can occur, or a non-ketotic hypoglycaemic coma may be precipitated.

Reagent strips which are to be used to measure blood glucose must be properly stored (sealed at room temperature) and correctly used. Even then, low levels may be inaccurately measured if the strips are more than 4 weeks old.

When insulin is required, the present preferred technique is to use a continuous insulin pump or drip infusion (Table 4.1) together with 1 litre of 5% dextrose every 8 hours (6.25 g/h). These administrations can be controlled by blood glucose estimations, or the proper use of reagent paper strips —Dextrostix or Boehringer. Allowances have to be made for the absorption of the soluble insulin onto any plastic tubing or syringe. Albumin- or gelatine-based plasma expanders may avoid absorption when passed through the system. In the presence of ketoacidosis preoperatively, there is a primary need to correct acid–base and electrolyte imbalance before anaesthesia is induced, and specialist advice may be required.

**Table 4.1**
*Regimens for diabetic patients*

| *Blood glucose (mmol/l)* | *Soluble insulin* |
|---|---|
| *Regimen 1:* Glucose or glucose/saline drip—variable syringe pump infusion of insulin (1 unit/ml solution) | |
| <4 | 0.5 units/h |
| 4–15 | 2.0 units/h |
| >15 | 4.0 units/h |
| >20 | Review |
| In resistant patients the rate may be doubled or quadrupled. | |
| *Regimen 2:* Glucose + insulin drip at basic fluid requirement rate | |
| <4 | 8 units/l |
| 5–15 | 16 units/l (start with 16 units/l) |
| >15 | 32 units/l |
| >20 | Review |
| Measure blood glucose every 2 hours until stable, then every 6 hours. | |

Control of acidosis and dehydration is a minimum requirement with very urgent surgery. As the use of hypertonic solution in patients who are already hyperosmolar may be hazardous, bicarbonate is now only used if the pH is less than 7.1. Lactate solutions (Ringer's) are unsuitable in such cases. Up to 8 units of insulin per hour may be required in the presence of ketoacidosis (0.1 u/kg). Preoperative anxiety is adrenergic and therefore cuts off insulin and may lead to increased blood sugar levels. Postoperatively, if a patient has received insulin by infusion he will have an increased demand for his diabetic-controlling drug for a period. Any patient who has diminished oral intake or nausea, after operations on the mouth for example, must receive continued care. Hypoxia, stress or shock causes lactic acidosis to which patients on older drugs, such as biguanides, are more prone. Such incidents should be reported to the physician in charge of the diabetic patient. Whatever the regimen, the anaesthetist's aim is to prevent a dangerous hypoglycaemia and to avoid the malnutrition to which a diabetic is prone as this aggravates the normal catabolic response to an operation. The method is to maintain carbohydrate and insulin availability throughout, while monitoring the blood glucose levels assiduously.

## Metabolic balance

Metabolic support for the young or old cannot be determined by a simple fixed rule; only guidelines are possible. One can be reasonably accurate in predicting metabolic reaction for the young fit patient, but not for the elderly or diseased. Indeed, tolerance to surgical trauma will be limited in most patients over 65 years of age, as more than 75% of them are affected by one or more chronic diseases. Changes in their endocrine response or physiological regulation are not apparent. For example, arterial pH is not changed with advanced age, although the rate of adjustment to basal levels is slower following displacement. In essence, all older patients must be treated within contracted margins of safety.

The old have less total body water and a smaller proportion of it is intracellular (approximately one-quarter of the body weight is a lower limit figure for females):

$$\frac{body\ weight}{4} = intracellular\ water$$

*Example:*

$$\frac{60}{4}\ kg = 15\ kg\ or\ litres$$

The daily need for each litre of intracellular water is as follows:

420 joules
(100 calories)
3 g protein
100 ml water
2 mmol potassium
3 mmol sodium

*or*

$$\text{body weight} \times \text{(kg)} \begin{cases} 105 \text{ joules (25 calories) available} \\ \quad \text{in 6 g of carbohydrate} \\ 25 \text{ ml water} \\ 0.75 \text{ g protein} \\ 0.75 \text{ mmol sodium} \\ 0.5 \text{ mmol potassium} \end{cases} \begin{array}{c} \text{daily} \\ \text{for} \\ \text{females} \end{array}$$

Nutrition can be seriously upset in the elderly coming up to an operation and it is a debatable point as to whether parenteral feeding will decrease mortality. Intravenous feeding requires exact control and cannot be undertaken lightly. If the measurement of the need and levels is faulty, complications are common. Thus, excess carbohydrate will produce extra carbon dioxide, which requires changed ventilation; fat may diminish defences against infection; and amino acids can alter levels of consciousness. All these incidents are more likely to occur in the older patient. Enteral or parenteral feeding should be applied preoperatively to the undernourished if there is time, and postoperatively beyond 4 or 5 days if oral intake is clearly going to be unsatisfactory (see Chapter 8).

Severe starvation with hypoproteinaemia and oedema, while significantly decreasing intracellular water, grossly expands the extracellular fluid and total body water. Similarly, chronic disease of the heart, kidneys and liver, with elevated levels of aldosterone, produces a disproportionate increase in extracellular water. Together with these changes, the total exchangeable potassium is reduced, while sodium remains stable.

Whereas a calculation of maintenance therapy based on the total intracellular water is a sound principle, it is more difficult to predict the elderly patient's metabolic reaction to trauma. Although their endocrine response may be normal, their tolerance to trauma is limited by their degenerative condition

—acidosis, hypoxia, hypercarbia or bacterial toxaemia can be overwhelming due to the patient's diminished functional reserve. Thus, limited cardiac reserve will make excessive administration of sodium or water intolerable. The additional energy requirement, due to restlessness, agitation, fever and wound repair, can be considerable. In a debilitated patient, glycogen stores may be exhausted and fat depleted. Lean tissue, as the only remaining source, may be being used at a rate of 2 kg per day. In such a case intravenous feeding is essential, although this must be undertaken with caution due to the hazard of excessive fluid being administered in an attempt to reach the caloric requirement.

The administration of quantities of fluid and electrolytes which would be appropriate to a young patient may be both unnecessary and detrimental to the old. Thus, a small old lady would require little more than half the usual daily requirement of the young adult. An underestimate of the deficit and frequent re-evaluation of the requirement are therefore of prime importance to avoid overexpansion of body fluid to the point of danger. It is clear that in older patients, cases of disturbance of expanded body fluid outnumber those cases in which contraction is predominant. In the wasted and debilitated old patient, a chronic, symptomless condition, precipitated by stress, is 'essential hyponatraemia'. It needs no treatment and is an expression of diminished reserve which requires careful administration of appropriate amounts of water and sodium. Otherwise, dilutional hyponatraemia, due to excessive crystalloid administration and water intoxication, will become evident quickly because it is related to the rate of change.

## Blood

Approximately 10% of aged patients have some anaemia, and blood volume studies years ago suggest that hypovolaemia was once commonplace. This is most related to the state of hydration; haemoconcentration from fasting can commonly be misleading. The viscosity of blood may be a crucial factor in its adequate flow and this is another important element in the amount of hydration or in the rarer polycythaemia. Once the patient has lost a certain amount of fat, the blood volume (in ml/kg) will rise—100 ml/kg is acceptable in thin patients, 70 ml/kg in the obese.

The blood volume of the aged is approximately 7% of the body weight, and plasma and erythrocytes are related to the extracellular water and body cell mass. While a blood loss of 30% is usually needed to cause serious hypotension, vasoconstriction and anaemia, smaller losses may produce these responses in the aged. Also, brain and heart blood flow compensation may be ineffective and deterioration of vital organs may rapidly ensue.

Coagulation problems are not frequent in the elderly, except with liver or blood diseases. A correct use of blood products will rectify most conditions. When there is severe jaundice it is likely that kidney function may be impaired and the patient will require frusemide or mannitol administration. It is necessary for vitamin K to be administered to those with jaundice, and coagulation studies must be done on these patients as well as on those who have any evidence of a tendency to bleed. Sickle cell testing of the races at risk is essential in the elderly, even more than in the young, as the old are more likely to suffer from the crisis-creating conditions of hypothermia, hypotension and hypoxia. Death in older sickle cell patients is more commonly due to thrombosis or embolism, rather than to the infections of which the young die.

## Miscellany

In considering the alimentary system the condition of the patient's teeth is of importance as it is related to airway management. In some instances, full dentures or mock-plates may be retained to facilitate better airways management. To prevent aspiration problems, it may be wise to administer antacids, metrocolpromide, ranitidine or cimetidine as indicated and, of course, gastric intubation and aspiration should be undertaken to alleviate any bowel obstruction.

Stomach content is of grave concern at all times, due to the hazard of aspiration. Hiatus hernias and oesophageal pouches are of particular concern, together with any form of obstruction, organic or functional. The patient's joints should be inspected carefully for mobility. The accessibility of veins and the presence or absence of pressure sores should be observed. Also, false eyes, limbs, joints or breasts are more likely to be present in the elderly and should be taken into account as potential hazards. In the elderly the site of the operation must be carefully marked as patients may be unreliable witnesses under medication or stress preoperatively and direct questions may then be unhelpful.

Today, monoamine oxidase inhibitors are less commonly used for treating depression. These should be withdrawn over a period of 2 weeks to minimise the risk of severe hypertension, pyrexia and convulsions which can occur due to the inhibitors' interaction with essential vasopressors or narcotics. Their replacements, the tricyclic antidepressants, will cause both anticholinergic and adrenergic potentiation, but it is not essential to withdraw them.

Other dangers of drug interactions lie with anticoagulants, antidiabetic therapy and antiparkinsonism drugs, all of which must be watched for, particularly in the elderly.

## Psychological care

Anaesthetists should become familiar with the simplest abbreviated mental tests. Aged patients who are more liable to mental problems are those who have previously been under psychiatric care, chronic alcoholics, the suicidal or those who appear to be unconcerned about their condition. Sudden uncooperativeness, suspicion, hostility, resentment, or evident argumentativeness and repetitive talk may be associated with poor memory and decreased intellect caused by a brain disorder.

The patient can only be calm when she or he believes that the recommended procedure is being done to improve their quality of life, or to find a means of doing so. Suspicion and misinformation are rife, so it is ideal to have a previous patient who has been successfully treated, to relate the experience to a new patient. Nurses and other staff can do a great deal to allay worries if they can be patient and reinforce information in the repetitious way which may be required. In the author's experience, older patients are often happier to receive author-itative instructions, and to carry them out, than are questioning younger patients. For the confused or demented, the same fulsome explanation and approach should be used, as it is never possible to define the exact degree of understanding. In these patients, of course, the consent signature will have to be obtained from a guardian or relative.

## Nervous system

A diagnosis of central nervous or neuromuscular disease makes the choice of conduction anaesthesia and the use of relaxants less straightforward. The efficacy of these methods must be balanced against the chance of medico-legal claims which may be made with a possible coincidental exacerbation of the disease. However, if a conduction block (or relaxants) is clearly the best form of anaesthesia, its use should not be avoided. No matter how grave the risk of operative death, anaesthesia should not be refused if there is a chance of improving the quality of life, and if the patient accepts that risk.

## Testing autonomic reflexes

Symptoms of autonomic neuropathy are vague but a battery of tests has been devised to show the abnormality. The simpler bedside tests are based on cardiovascular reflexes, using heart rate changes with a Valsalva manoeuvre, spontaneous or deep breathing, or blood pressure changes with standing or during sustained exercise, for example hand grip. There are many more cardiovascular reflex tests and tests of sweating, bladder, bowel and pupil function, some using drugs or biochemical analysis. Some tests look at failure of a part of a system, but a few gross non-invasive tests requiring little physical and mental effort on behalf of the elderly patients are most practical.

1. Heart rate is recorded by electrocardiogram in a seated subject, breathing in and out slowly once every 10 seconds for three or four times. The minimum and maximum rate differences are equal to or greater than 15 beats per minute normally, but equal to or less than 10 beats per minute with autonomic failure.

2. Heart rate is recorded by electrocardiogram in a subject lying for 2 minutes for a few beats before standing, until about

40 beats after standing. The shortest R–R interval (about the 15th beat) and the longest R–R interval (about the 30th beat) after beginning to stand are measured and the maximum-to-minimum ratio is calculated. The ratio is normally equal to or greater than 1.04, and abnormally equal to or less than 1.0. These heart rate tests are independent of resting rates but invalid if ectopic beats are recorded.

3. When a patient stands autonomic failure is indicated if the systolic blood pressure drop is equal to or greater than 30 mmHg. This drop, however, may be due to hypovolaemia or any of many drugs and, conversely, hypotension may not occur in congestive cardiac failure or nephrotic syndrome.

Skin wrinkling reduction, lower body negative pressure application and vasomotor tests (hot and cold responses) plus finger blood flow) have also been used in the elderly to test autonomic system integrity.

In summary, of the investigatons mentioned, the $FEV_1$ systolic blood pressure and creatinine clearance, together with the glucose tolerance, show most correlation with perioperative survival.

Attempts to correct heart failure, chronic bronchitis, diabetic conditions, dehydration and angina and to provide maximum attention to emergency patients with hypovolaemia, hypothermia, malnourishment or electrolyte imbalance, are not refinements but vital preoperative preparation for old patients. As previously indicated, such attention must never be rushed or limited for the sake of convenience.

## Premedication

The purposes of premedication are to assist in induction and maintenance of anaesthesia, reduce airway secretion and provide euphoria. In modern anaesthesia the dominant aim is to relieve anxiety, through the personal reassurance and explanation provided by the anaesthetist on her or his preoperative visit to the patient. Such a visit is essential, not only for the assessment and preparation already described, but also for psychological purposes, and management of the anaesthetic and postoperative period will be much easier for the trouble taken. If the visit is on the evening before the operation, it is possible to ensure that the patient gets a proper night's rest. For this, it is essential to choose a sedative or tranquilliser which will have the minimum side-effect or interaction with any drug which will subsequently be necessary.

It may be wise to ensure that there is no extension of the drugs utilised for anaesthesia into the pre- or postoperative period because only during the actual anaesthetic are patients under the direct control of the anaesthetist. Thus, there should be little place for ataractics or neuroleptics preoperatively, although their use during the operation may be expected to extend postoperatively. Indeed, the simplest of sedatives, chlormethiozole or chloralhydrate, and anxiolytic hypnotics, such as temazepam, triazolam, or oxazepam which can now replace the older pure tranquillisers, produce little anaesthetic potentiation or vasomotor depression. All these drugs can be given orally, eliminating the need for injection. There is no evidence that oral administration, compared with injection of premedication, changes the amount or acidity of the stomach contents.

Except in the presence of pain preoperatively, the routine use of narcotics is no longer justifiable. The unwanted effects of vomiting, nausea and respiratory depression are important, and the last-mentioned can be extremely dangerous in the sick elderly. This recommendation is reinforced by the fact that the once routine use of anticholinergic drugs (which could act as antidotes to some of the narcotic side-effects) is no longer advised preoperatively. The side-effects of the anticholinergic drugs themselves are unacceptable, and the claimed benefits are unnecessary or illtimed.

Excess salivary and bronchial secretions are a rare consequence of modern anaesthetics and the drying effects of the preoperative administration of atropine lead to sore throats and thickening of secretions, together with palpitations which can be most uncomfortable. Rarely has atopine been incriminated in the old as a cause of coma, parotitis or *Monilia* infections, Hyoscine, on the other hand, is long acting and frequently produces restlessness and confusion in the elderly, or even respiratory depression. Their elimination as routine premedication would obviate the problem of anticholinergic drugs with narrow-angle glaucoma or prostatism. When there is vagal overactivity, either preoperatively or due to any of the common parasympathetic stimuli from agents and methods of anaesthesia, the timing of the anticholinergic drug is so crucial that the intravenous route should be used. Digitalis, anticoagulants, antidepressants, bronchodilators, and antihypertensives may be continued preoperatively. One should stop monoamine oxidase inhibitors, boost steroids and check diabetic control.

The longer acting benzodiazepines—diazepam, lorazepam, nitrazepam and flunitrazepam—are all less satisfactory than the short acting—oxazepam, temazepam and triazolam—in that they may cause some respiratory depression and anaesthetic and relaxant interaction through their overlapping effect (Table 4.2). The same may be said of earlier tranquillisers, such as meprobramate and chlordiazepoxide. All benzodiazepines produce amnesia earlier and longer in the old, with a possible consequent loss of contact and confusion perioperatively. For old patients pethidine and promethazine are still popular premedicants with some anaesthetists, but in reduced doses they are of little value.

### Table 4.2
*Benzodiazepines (oral administration)*

| Drug | Mean half-life (hours) | Range (hours) | Dose for >65 years old (mg) |
|------|------------------------|---------------|------------------------------|
| *Long acting* | | | |
| Diazepam | 32 | 14–61 | 5 |
| Lorazepam | 13 | 8–24 | 2 |
| Nitrazepam | 28 | 18–38 | 5 |
| Flunitrazepam | 15 | 9–25 | 1 |
| *Short acting* | | | |
| Oxazepam | 8 | 3–14 | 25 |
| Temazepam | 8 | 6–9 | 20 |
| Triazolam | 4 | 3–5 | 0.25 |

**Further reading**

*Assessment*
Caird F.L. (1973). Problems of interpretation of laboratory findings in the old. *Brit. Med. J*; **4**:68.
Cooperman H. *et al.* (1978). Cardiovascular risk factors in patients with peripheral vascular disease. *Surg*; **84**:505.

Del Guercio L.R.M., Cohn J.D. (1980). Monitoring operative risk in the elderly. *J. Am. Med. Assoc*; **243**:1350.

Denham M. *et al.* (1984). Value of routine chest radiography in an acute geriatric unit. *Brit. Med. J*; **288**:1726.

Denham M.J., Jefferys P.M. (1972). Routine mental testing in the elderly. *Mod. Geriatrics*; **2**:275.

Domaingue C.M. *et al.* (1982). Cardiovascular risk factors in patients with vascular disease. *Anaesth. Int. Care*; **10**:234.

Foex P. (1978). Preoperative assessment of patients with cardiac disease. *Brit. J. Anaesth*; **50**:15.

Goldman L. (1983). Cardiac risks and complications of non-cardiac operations. *Int. Med.*; **98**:504.

Gudwin A.L. *et al.* (1968). Estimation of ventricular mixing volume for prediction of operative mortality in the elderly. *Ann. Surg*; **168**:183.

Haljamae H. *et al.* (1982). Preanaesthetic evaluation of the female geriatric patient with hip fracture. *Acta Anaesthesiol. Scand*; **26**:393.

Keats A.S. (1978). The A.S.A. classification of physical status — a recaptitulation. *Anesthesiol*; **49**:233.

Lindau S. *et al.* (1969). Mental and functional status in the elderly: relationship to blood gas and pH levels. *J. Am. Geriatr. Soc*; **17**:924.

Martin V.C. (1977). Hypoxaemia in elderly patients suffering from fractured neck of femur. *Anaesth*; **32**:852.

McNaulty J. et al. (1978). A prospective study of sudden death in high risk bundle branch block. *New Engl. J. Med*; **299**:209.

Maseri A. *et al.* (1964). Clinical applications of radiocardiography. *Acta Med. Scand*; **176**:169.

Milne J.S., Williamson J. (1972). Respiratory function tests in older people. *Clin. Sci*; **42**:371.

Morris J.F. *et al.* (1971). Sprirometric standards for healthy non-smoking adults. *Am. Rev. Resp. Dis*; **103**:37.

Pastereo J.D. *et al.* (1978). The risk of advanced heart block in surgical patients with right bundle branch block and left axis deviation. *Circulation*; **57**:677.

Phillips G., Tomlin P.J. (1977). Arterial oxygen tensions in elderly and in injured elderly patients. *Brit. J. Anaesth*; **49**:514.

Seymour D.G. *et al.* (1983). The role of routine preoperative electrocardiographs in the elderly surgical patient. *Age and Ageing*; **12**:97.

Steen P.A. *et al.* (1978). Myocardial reinfarction after anesthesia and surgery. *J. Am. Med. Assoc*; **239**:2566.

Tachakra S.S., Sevitt S. (1975). Hypoemia after fractures. *J. Bone & Jt. Surg*; **57**:197.

Tarhans S. *et al.* (1972). Myocardial reinfarction after general anesthesia. *J. Am. Med. Assoc*; **220**:1451.

Taylor I.C., Stout, R.W. (1983). The significance of cardiac arrhythmias in the aged. *Age and Ageing*; **12**:21.

Wang K.C., Howland W.G. (1958). Cardiac and pulmonary evaluation in elderly patients before elective surgical operations. *J. Am. Med. Assoc*; **166**:993.

Ward R.J. *et al.* (1966). Effect of posture on normal arterial blood gas tension in the aged. *Geriatrics*; **21**:139.

Wijesurendra R.J. *et al.* (1981). Incidence of concurrent disease in the surgical population of a tertiary care hospital. *Can. Anaesth. Soc. J.*; **28**:67.

Wilson L.A. *et al.* (1973). Brief assessment of the mental state in geriatric domicilary practice; the usefulness of the mental status questionnaire. *Age and Ageing*; **2**:92.

*Preparation*

Castleden C.M. *et al.* (1977). Increased sensitivity to nitrazepam in old age. *Brit. Med. J*; **1**:10.

Chadwick D.A. (1973). Reducing anaesthetic risks for the geriatric surgical patient. *Geriatrics*; **28**:108.

Cook P.J. *et al.* (1984). Diazepam tolerance: effect of age, regular sedation and alcohol. *Brit. Med. J*; **289**:351.

Edwards R. *et al.* (1977). Acute hypocapnoeic hypokalemia — an iatrogenic anaesthetic complication. *Anesth. Analg*; **56**:786.

Egbert L.D. *et al.* (1964). Reduction of postoperative pain by management and instruction of patients. *New Eng. J. Med*; **270**:825.

Foex P., Prys-Roberts C. (1974). Anaesthesia and the hypertensive patient. *Brit. J. Anaesth*; **46**:575.

Fowler N.O. (1981). Noncardiac surgery in the elderly patient with heart disease. *Cardiovasc. Clin. (US)*; **12**:211.

Goldman L., Caldera D.L. (1979). Risks of general anesthesia and elective operation in the hypertensive patients. *Anesthesiol*; **50**:285.

Gothard J.W., Branthwaite M.A., (1979). Cardiac pacemaker insertion: a study of the anaesthetic and postoperative complications. *Anaesth*; **34**:269.

Greenblatt D.J. *et al.* (1984). Effect of age, gender and obesity on midazolam kinetics. *Anesthesiol*; **61**:27.

Hickler R.B., Van Dam L.D. (1970). Hypertension. *Anesthesiol*; **33**:214.

Inglis J.M. (1967). Premedication in geriatric patients. *Geriatrics*; **22 Sept**:1150.

Johnson J.C. (1953). The medical evaluation and management of the elderly surgical patient. *J. Am. Geriatr. Soc*; **31**:621.

Kul J. *et al.* (1978). Prophylaxis of post operative p.e. and d.v.t. by low dose heparin. *Lancet*; **1**:1115.

Macdonald T.B. *et al.* (1983). Coronary care in the elderly. *Age and Ageing*; **12**:17.

Michel L.J. *et al.* (1983). Preoperative prophylactic digitalization of patients with coronary artery disease — a randomised echocardiographic and hemodynamic study. *Anesth. Analg*; **62**:865.

Miller R.R. *et al.* (1975). Propranolol withdrawal rebound phenomenon. *New Engl. J. Med*; **293**:416.

Negus D. *et. al.* (1980). Ultra-low dose intravenous heparin in the prevention of post-operative deep-vein thrombosis. *Lancet*; **i**: 891

Ngai S.H. (1972). Parkinsonism, Levodopa and anesthesia. *Anesthesiol*; **37**:344.

Plumpton F.S. *et al.* (1969). Corticosteroid treatment and surgery. The management of steroid cover. *Anaesth*; **24**:12.

Prys-Roberts C. (1979). Hypertension and anaesthesia — fifty years on. *Anesthesiol*; **50**:251.

Risbo A., Schmidt J.F. (1983). Per oral diazepam compared with parenteral morphine/scopolamine with regard to gastric contents. *Acta Anaesthesiol. Scand*; **27**:165.

Rodstein M., Oei L. (1979). Cardiovascular side effects of long term therapy with tricyclic antidepressants in the aged. *J. Am. Geriatr. Soc*; **27**:231.

Roger R. L. *et. al.* (1985). Abstention from cigarette smoking improves cerebral perfusion among elderly chronic smokers. *J. Am. Med. Assoc*; **253**: 2970.

Roy W.L. *et al.* (1979). Myocardial ischaemia during noncardiac surgical procedures in patients with coronary artery disease. *Anesthesiol*; **51**:393.

Salem M.G., Ahearn R.S. (1984). The effect of atrophine and glycopyrrolate on intraocular pressure in anaesthetised elderly patients. *Anaesth*; **39**:809.

Simon A.B. (1977). Perioperative management of the pacemaker patient. *Anesthesiol*; **46**:127.

Smyth N.P.D. *et al.* (1974). The pacemaker patient and the electromagnetic environment. *J. Am. Med. Assoc*; **227**:1412.

Swift C.G. *et al.* (1981). The effect of ageing on measured responses to single doses of oral temazepam. *Brit. J. Clin. Pharmacol*; **11**:413.

Wynards J.E. (1976). Anesthesia for patients with heart block and artificial cardiac pacemakers. *Anesth. Anal*; **56**:626.

# CHAPTER 5

# Anaesthetic management

> The margin of safety (or we might call it the 'allowance for carelessness') is much less in an old person than in a robust young one.
>
> *H.R. Griffith*

## Preliminaries

It is essential in all cases to ensure that the correct patient has the correct operation, but this is particularly important in the case of the elderly because they often cannot communicate well. Wrist-band identification and skin marking of the operation site are mandatory. The anaesthetist and surgeon must recognise the patients and be familiar with their conditions. If, on arrival in the operating theatre, the patient complains of further symptoms, such as breathlessness, chest pain or weakness, the doctors involved must take time to assess their importance and, if necessary, postpone the operation for further investigation or for treatment of recent serious complications. The risks of what the Americans call 'rush' surgery are only acceptable for life-endangering hypoxia ischaemia or bleeding.

The principles of anaesthesia for the elderly, even more rigorously applied to the aged, are that the minimum amount of agents should be given with the greatest of care. The same principles of anaesthesia apply to neonates, but the assiduous preparation and expert experience of those handling the very young are rarely apparent with the aged. Encyclopaedic knowledge is far less useful than finesse, with gentleness of techniques and conscientious attention to details of observation and management. Meticulous attention on the part of anaesthetists is best achieved by what Dr Peter Dinnick calls 'watch keeping ability'—that is, a constant scanning of variables is taught so that it becomes second nature to have a form of mental alarm clock to pick up changes in the patient's state. The published experience of different forms of anaesthesia are mostly from proponents of a particular choice which they administer with special care. The tendency is to rely most on general anaesthesia because it is always applicable and is therefore a loadstone to trainees who handle most of the elderly cases.

There are very few proven specific age-dependent differences in the response to drugs used by anaesthetists. Nevertheless, there are exaggerated and delayed normal responses in many instances which are clinically important. The patient adequately prepared psychologically, supplemented if need be by sedation with a hypnotic, should arrive in the operating theatre undepressed and unstressed.

Induction of anaesthesia should be accomplished in as comfortable a way as possible; this begins with the patient being allowed to adopt whatever posture he or she finds most suitable—sitting or flexed. This may entail support of the back or legs. There should be no haste because the initial and full effect of drugs is always liable to be prolonged. Any form of conduction anaesthesia should be carried out with a great deal of explanation to the patient concerning its undertaking as the procedure advances.

There are some routines for all patients which must never be neglected in the old. It is necessary first to place a needle or cannula in an arm vein or to verify carefully the satisfactory state of an infusion already in place. Pressure over the usual site of a vein in the presence of oedema may well facilitate venepuncture when it appears impossible. For the most ill patients, movement from the bed to the operating table should be before anaesthetic induction. For those in pain, an intravenous injection of narcotic may be required before movement. All movements must be gentle. A preliminary heart rate and arterial pressure recording should be made. In those at extra risk any other helpful monitoring system should be provided before induction, for example ECG, arterial pressure. After induction, when longer-acting relaxants are to be used, application of a nerve stimulator before paralysis is most helpful to define the supramaximal current for the chosen sites of the electrodes. Temperature monitoring by thermocouple (taped to the skin under gamgee) in nasopharynx, oesophagus or rectum, should be used when the operation is likely to be prolonged.

**Induction**

If bradycardia indicates that a patient has strong vagal tone
and if parasympathomimetic drugs are to be used, for example
suxamethonium, halothane or cyclopropane, atropine should
be administered intravenously, under ECG control when the
blood pressure is low. It must be remembered that the raised
intraocular pressure this may cause can induce acute glaucoma
or vitreous loss in certain patients. Some prefer glycopyrronium bromide for its stronger tonic effect on the oesophageal
cardiac spincter and for its prolonged action, but it has not yet
completed a 'test of time'. In the elderly there will more
frequently be a longer arm-to-brain circulation time and
consequently the onset of action of an injected drug will be
delayed in a considerable proportion of patients. This may
affect the rate of onset of an opiate analgesic which is
frequently given at this point, but not as obviously as it will
affect the hypnotic drug that may be injected. Circulation time
is indeed a crucial factor in the onset of action of thiopentone
and other intravenous induction drugs, while the volume into
which they are distributed will determine their maximum
action.

Two other conditions which are clearly related to the need
for a reduced dose of any induction agent are anaemia and
uraemia—conditions common in the elderly. If a fixed rate of
injection is used, it is likely that there will be considerable risk
of giving an overdose which may cause respiratory arrest or
severe cardiovascular depression. The usual method—taught
and studied—of giving repeated increments at intervals of less
than a minute, or an infusion, will always result in an
overdose—the older the patient, the more serious. For this
reason it is sensible to dilute all intravenous induction agents,
to give a minimum calculated dose in a bolus injection, and to
wait at least 60 seconds before any additional injection. The
end-point before unconsciousness may best be taken as a
voluntary action of the patient such as counting or hand raising.
Lash reflexes and responses to painful stimuli may be retained
much beyond unconsciousness.

Because of the slow and enhanced response and greater
variability, especially after premedication, any judgement of
the dose is imprecise (Fig. 5.1; Table 5.1). If the condition of

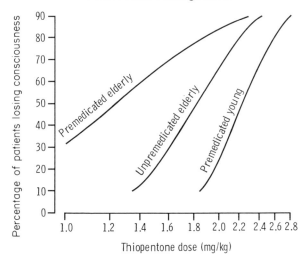

**Fig. 5.1** The bolus dose of 2.5% of thiopentone intravenously related to the age and premedication (morphine 5 mg) required to produce loss of consciousness.

the patient, or the inaccessibility of a vein, indicates it, an inhalation induction should be chosen without compunction. Properly undertaken, this is not unpleasant and is more controllable than intravenous induction. Because of the changes of pulmonary function there may, however, be a slower change of alveolar and arterial blood levels of the inhaled anaesthetic, particularly in the presence of increased lung residual volume and emphysema. When such slowness prolongs the second stage, or fearfulness occurs during the application of the mask causing a stormy beginning of anaesthesia, it is wise to switch to an intravenous or intramuscular agent.

With experience, and some skill, a combination of intravenous and inhalation induction is best of all. After a very small bolus dose of intravenous agent, an oxygen-enriched inhalation agent is applied, with hypnotic suggestion, as the mask is lowered onto the patient's face.

With a 'crash' induction when the hypnotic is contributing to unawareness of the intubation, a larger dose is required. Because of the hypotension due to peripheral vasodilatation caused by intravenous induction agents, a 'preloading' fluid infusion may help. An overdose in the elderly, particularly those with reduced plasma protein leaving unbound drug,

**Table 5.1**

*Bolus doses of induction agents to produce loss of consciousness in the elderly and aged with light premedication (morphine or benzodiazepine)*

| Induction agent | In 20 ml of saline | 65–75 years (mg/kg) | 75+ (mg/kg) |
|---|---|---|---|
| Thiopentone | 150 mg (0.75%) | 1.5 | 0.75 |
| Methohexitone | 50 mg (0.25%) | 0.5 | 0.25 |
| Etomidate | 20 mg (0.1%) | 0.2 | 0.1 |
| Ketamine | 100 mg (0.5%) | 1 | 0.5 |
| Midazolam | 4 mg (0.02%) | 0.04 | 0.02 |

*Note.* A bolus injection should be followed by an interval of at least 1 min. Use subjective signs of unconsciousness.

causes a more profound cardiovascular and central nervous system effect. Except in 'crash' induction, the immediate continuation from the intravenous induction to a slow introduction of the inhalation agents should be routine. This unhurried induced unconsciousness enables a more likely initiation of the individual's homoeostatic mechanisms to counter the drug effects, it gives an opportunity to assess any problems with airway management, and contributes to the reduction of the required relaxant dosage by eliminating reflexes.

Any slowed circulation will also lead to delayed onset of action of relaxants. With suxamethonium, muscle fasciculation may be late or minimal and, if this is unappreciated, it may lead to a second unnecessary dose. Good airway management and manipulation of a face mask in the old require considerable experience. Strong mandibular traction by the hands of the anaesthetist is not always fruitful, neither may be an oropharyngeal airway placed before reflexes are fully obtuded. Extension of the neck with one hand on the patient's forehead, application of the face mask with the thumb and forefinger of the other hand with the other three fingers of the same hand cradling the patient's jaw as it relaxes, is a technique most likely to provide the best airway control. A child's airway or bite block to part the lips, full dentures, a dental prop or stent mould, or a latex rubber nasopharyngeal tube may all be of use at times. The mask fit is often a source of difficulty and all sizes and shapes should be available. The very large, infolded edge type of mask (Everseal) may on occasion be successful. In some instances an oropharyngeal block type of airway or direct attachment to one or two nasopharyngeal tubes with a pack in the mouth is useful. With kyphosis, a double pillow may be required throughout anaesthesia. During the induction period the anaesthetist should at all times occupy the mind of the patient with soothing encouraging talk. He should placate the patient as required while repeating preoperative instructions concerning chest care and activity postoperatively, because cerebral imprinting during induction can reinforce memorisation.

The original intravenous route should contain a diaphragm or tap system and be kept patent, if there is no continuous infusion. The sequence of a butterfly needle for the original injection followed by cannulation with a plastic catheter is advantageous in that the fine needle causes little pain and the cannula can be placed when the veins have become distended or dilated. The choice of drip site is important for the elderly, who may later become confused, so it should be chosen and fixed with great care. The dilution of induction agents should considerably reduce the venous thrombosis which can occur commonly in elderly patients after injections. This is most obvious in the case of peripheral vein injection of diazepam, which is followed by an increasingly high incidence of venous thrombosis in old patients (see Fig. 3.3 in Chapter 3). Diazepam mixed with soyabean oil and water (Diazemuls) may overcome this to a great extent. Small doses of diazepam, ketamine or midazolam may be given as a preliminary to moving patients into an operating theatre to avoid the danger of movement after anaesthesia has begun, or for positioning patients for regional anaesthesia.

In seriously ill patients whose cardiovascular condition is considered critical, it has been suggested that induction may be undertaken more safely with these agents rather than the usual induction agents. Older anaesthetists may prefer cyclopropane for anaesthesia induction in shocked patients. However, provided the induction agents are used with much circumspection, there would appear to be little to choose between them, and no one agent has yet been shown clearly to be preferable. A considerable number of elderly patients will, after induction anaesthesia, be subject to bladder catheterisation. This is best done using full aseptic precautions within the theatre and is invaluable for urinary output monitoring perioperatively. A small-diameter (12 FG) siliconised balloon catheter (Foley) is preferable.

## Endotracheal intubation

The usual mandatory and relative indications apply to intubation of elderly patients. To these are added the need (as with infants) for airway control and assisted and controlled ventilation which is beneficial in extremes of age for all but the most short minor operations. However, an insistence on intubation for all young and old patients is unreasoned. Small doses of intravenous induction agents, without a preliminary narcotic or subsequent inhalation agent, produce a level of unconsciousness which is insufficient to prevent response to the stimuli of laryngoscopy and intubation. In any lightly anaesthetised patient, such a stress response causes an increase in heart rate and blood pressure, and with cardiovascular disease, grave dysrhythmia or myocardial ischaemia. Many methods have been tried to prevent this, but to ensure a moderate depth of anaesthesia, and intravenous fentanyl or alfentanil appear to be the most practical.

During anaesthesia, hypertension can be reduced by cautious increase of the concentration of a volatile halogenated anaesthetic agent or, rarely, by intravenous sodium nitroprusside or nitroglycerine. Forceful movement, especially flexion of an arthritic neck (Fig. 5.2a) can be very damaging, and preoperative mobility estimates or cervical vertebral x-rays are only rough guides to this problem. Over-vigorous extension of the neck may obstruct the blood supply to the brain, especially where there is basilar artery insufficiency. Cervical manipulative techniques can cause reflex spasm of the posterior cerebellar or vertebral arteries in the presence of abnormal anatomy or disease (Fig. 5.2b). Narrowing of these arteries occurs with extension and rotation of the neck. In one study, forceful turning of the head to one side decreased the flow through the opposite carotid artery by over a quarter. Such a positional test, if maintained for several seconds, may indicate those at risk if dizziness, nystagmus or dysarthria occurs. Neck position during laryngoscopy may obstruct the neck veins, or

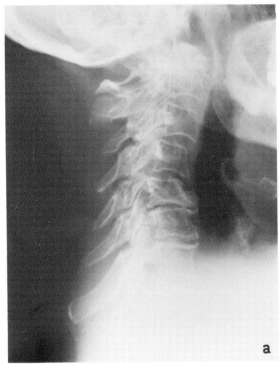

**Fig. 5.2(a)** A lateral x-ray of the cervical spine showing erosion of the odontoid peg and subluxation of C3 on C4 and C4 on C5. There are degenerative changes also at C5/C6 and C6/C7 levels.

the period of apnoea during direct vision of the larynx may be so prolonged that the $Pa_{CO_2}$ rises markedly. The prevention is obvious, but in neurosurgery where controlled cerebral pressure is crucial, intravenous practalol and passive over-ventilation may also be utilised before intubation.

For the old, conscious intubation should be as readily used as it is for neonates; it is the best way of ensuring airway protection. With the correct choice of suitable patients, full explanation to obtain cooperation, and exceeding gentleness, it is highly successful. A local anaesthetic lozenge, local anaesthetic aerosol inhalation, topical anaesthetic applied progressively to the pharynx and glottic opening (Fig. 5.3), or a transtracheal injection may all help. Sudden vomiting or regurgitation may occur, so it should be possible to lower the

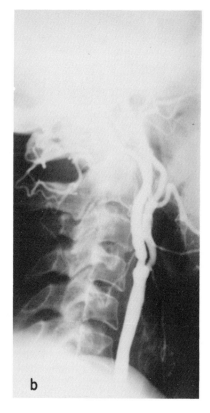

**Fig. 5.2(b)** A selective angiography of the left carotid artery shows 50% stenosis of the internal carotid artery just beyond its origin.

head of the patient and use suction promptly. The dosage of tropical anaesthesia should be carefully controlled and 2% lignocaine concentration is adequate $(3 \text{ mg/kg})^{-1}$. High-powered jet sprays are liable to cause strong stimuli and glottic closure, so that a malleable semisoft cannula with an attached syringe holding the calculated dose is preferable. The peak blood level after topical absorption occurs after 10 minutes and the toxic phenomena must be aborted rapidly.

Once intubation has been accomplished, immediate induction of anaesthesia can follow for patient comfort, and probably amnesia of the event. The air inflated endotracheal cuff distends with nitrous oxide loculation; this distention

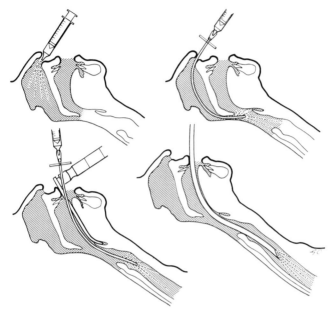

**Fig. 5.3** Progressive topical anaesthesia application (shaded area) for conscious endotracheal intubation.

must be reduced at intervals to prevent airway mucosal damage. If the cuff is inflated with pure nitrous oxide or saline, this problem does not arise.

For almost all operations on the bowel (and some others), a nasogastric tube is required. If the tube is *in situ* preoperatively, the fear that it may initiate regurgitation seems unfounded, provided it is aspirated and left open before anaesthesia. Much the greatest concern with regurgitation is the increased intragastric pressure which may be markedly and suddenly aggravated by respiratory obstruction. In most patients with a tube *in situ*, a rapid induction is indicated. The so-called 'crash' induction is a sequence of oxygen administration, cricoid pressure (Sellick manoeuvre), intravenous induction of anaesthesia and suxamethonium, and intubation and cuff inflation. This technique has now been widely practised for over 20 years. Although it must undoubtedly have prevented aspiration of stomach contents in many circumstances, it has created its own morbidity and mortality. In the old patient there is firstly the difficulty of estimating the required anaesthetic induction agent dose which, if excessive, as a bolus, may create severe cardiovascular collapse, particularly in those in incipient shock. The application of cricoid pressure is liable to vary greatly in its efficiency depending upon the assistants providing the help and their tuition and experience. When misapplied it may distort the direct laryngoscopic view and make intubation difficult, or it may fail to block the pharyngeal regurgitation.

In the case of failed intubation or aspiration, the regimes commonly activated in obstetric anaesthesia must be used routinely. The original description of the Sellick manoeuvre, using the index finger for pressure on the cricoid cartilage at the front and its centralisation with the thumb and third finger, is not always easy owing to the great variation of neck structures which exist. A straight compression, with three fingers of the assistant's hand palm down on the chest is more easily applied (Fig. 5.4).

If, after induction of anaesthesia and intubation, a Ryle or Levine tube is to be passed from the nose to the stomach, negotiation past the cricopharyngeal region is often difficult. Many methods of overcoming this have been described but the most successful is as follows.

Insert a well-lubricated nasogastric tube into the hypopharynx through the nose; lift the larynx off the posterior pharyngeal wall from the outside with one hand (Fig. 5.4), pass the tube into the upper oesophagus, and advance the tube to the stomach with an index finger in the pharynx to prevent the tube curling. It seems likely that the obstruction is not so much active cricopharyngeal sphincter closure as posterior displacement of the relaxed larynx or tube cuff blockage due to its distension of the soft posterior part of the trachea. The type of nasogastric tube does not seem material, and a size 12–16 gauge (French) is usually employed. Of course, in the very old, this manoeuvre must be carried out with an extra degree of gentleness so that the calcified cartilages of the larynx are not damaged. Blind passage of the tube past the nasopharyngeal angle must be cautious so that the mucous lining is not damaged or the tube passed into mediastinal tissue.

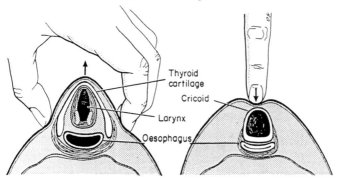

**Fig. 5.4** A transverse section of the neck when the oesophagus is being opened and closed by manipulation from the front.

## Regional anaesthesia

When conduction analgesia is to have a major role in the anaesthetic, it commences with the same monitoring requirements and an intravenous route being provided. The use of conduction analgesia should be widely encouraged because there is considerable evidence that the general morbidity is reduced in patients who can be managed in this way. This evidence concerns the strong nociceptive stimuli which produce many physiological changes presenting as surgical stress. If this stress is prevented, heart rate and pressure increases with associated myocardial ischaemia are reduced, postoperative hypoxaemia is less and briefer, gastrointestinal function and repair are better, deep vein thrombosis is less common, and many body reactions are muted. Because older patients are less able to withstand these changes, the benefits are obvious.

A block may be accomplished with a conscious patient when a full explanation and continued explanation of everything that follows is undertaken. Basic requirements are that the patient is willing to have a local anaesthetic, the technique is practical and adequate for the operation, and comfort can be ensured for the duration needed. Local analgesia can also be utilised with light forms of general anaesthesia or varying degrees of sedation, but then, and with unsupplemented blocks, optimal vigilance must be maintained. For infiltration and field or plexus blocks, the concentration of analgesic agents can usually be progressively reduced with advancing age. However, the reduction of volume does not seem as successful. The most common error is to allow insufficient time for the block to become fully effective. As explained in Chapter 1, the anatomy and bony landmarks in the elderly are advantageous for the accomplishment of these blocks.

The Bier intravenous regional block is also of considerable value, both for the upper and lower limbs. The agent preferred is a 0.5% or 0.25% lignocaine or prilocaine, rather than agents with extra toxicity due to strong protein binding. A small plastic cannula (rather than a needle) to give the drug, and a pneumatic exsanguinating device (rather than an Esmarch bandage) are preferable. The tourniquet should be properly applied and carefully checked at regular intervals. The use of a tourniquet for this or other reasons may be questioned because the vessels of old patients are fragile, prone to rupture and later liable to thrombus or inflammation. Tourniquet pressure should be just 10–20 mmHg above the systolic blood pressure, release should be staged, and the patient observed carefully during the release period. Refinements of the technique, such as confining a major part of the drug to the area of operation by the brief use of a secondary tourniquet during injection and the rapid release and reinflation of the tourniquet with the limb compressed to reduce back-bleeding, are helpful in some instances. Release of a tourniquet (as with unclamping the aorta in vascular surgery) causes a sudden reduction of peripheral resistance with a blood pressure fall, acidosis from accumulated lactate, and a rise in serum potassium. Clinically this is not often serious, but in the older patient it is more liable to precipitate a critical state and therefore requires special attention.

*Spinal block*

Epidural and subarachnoid anaesthesia have an important place in the management of elderly patients. The only absolute contraindications are patient refusal and infection in the proposed injection site, plus coagulation problems for epidural injections. Relative contraindications include central nervous disease, shock, septicaemia, obstructed bowel, concurrent drug administration which changes cardiovascular responses, and spinal deformity (Fig. 5.5). The common vital concern is the degree of preganglionic block of sympathetic nerves leading to

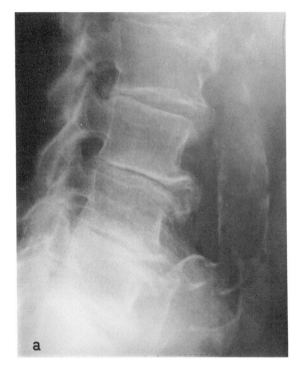

**Fig. 5.5(a)** A lumbar x-ray with a loss of disc space, reactive sclerosis and marginal osteophytosis. Heavy calcified aorta and iliac vessels.

peripheral vasodilatation and therefore hypotension. This hypotension may be countered by fluid infusion, by the cautious use of a vasopressor, e.g. ephedrine or methoxamine, and by assiduous prevention of impairment of venous return by vena caval occlusion, or by judicious adjustment of posture. The degree of hypotension depends on the level of the block, which usually must be above T10 for there to be any serious effect. In the old, reflex compensation for hypotension is inefficient. Hypotension may be faster in onset and more marked with spinal than with epidural block. If the block extends above T4, then cardiac accelerator nerves are affected and a slow pulse will result. When T1 level is affected, the patient may complain of numbness or tingling in the little finger. However, the respiratiory system is rarely seriously affected if the block is below C4, and the decrease of renal

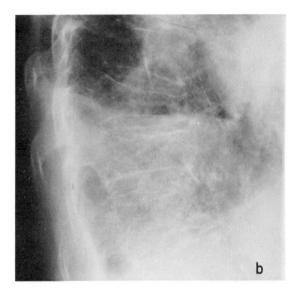

**Fig. 5.5(b)** Osteoporotic lower thoracic vertebrae with anterior wedging of T8 and T9 showing vertebral collapse.

function will be dependent on the degree of blood pressure drop.

In most spinal blocks there is sacral parasympathetic block but no vagal block. Sudden arterial hypotension from vaso-vagal reflexes with visceral manipulation is thus possible but uncommon in the aged and prevented with general anaesthesia. However, general anaesthesia in the presence of regional block may limit compensatory vasoconstriction in the unblocked area. Thus hypotension is more common in anaesthetised blocked patients.

To steer an old patient through a major operation using spinal block requires meticulous care and a cooperative surgeon, but it can be very rewarding. Subarachnoid single injection technique is aimed at producing the block of a calculated number of dermatomes which may be stimulated by the operation. As a guide, the important levels to remember are pubis L1, umbilicus T10, xiphisternum T6, and nipple line T4. The autonomic visceral supply is more complex, and the vagal supply will be unaffected by any appropriate block.

*Upper segmental nerve supply to abdominal viscera*
T6　　Stomach, spleen and pancreas

T7    Liver and gall bladder
T8    Adrenals
T9    Small bowel
T10   Uterus, testis, ovary, kidney and ureter
T11   Bladder, prostate and proximal large bowel
L1    Distal large bowel, including rectum

The level of subarachnoid block is slightly dependent on gravity (relative specific gravity of agent) and posture, but mostly on the volume of agent (plus barbotage). With bupivacaine, the level is slightly higher and the block onset faster and profounder with ageing. The level of block with epidural injection is dependent on the patient's height, obesity, volume of agent, site and force or rate of injection, plus direction of the needle bevel.* Therefore a continuous catheter technique with incremental injection offers greater control. There is argument as to whether a test dose is helpful, but 5 ml of 2% lignocaine with adrenaline 1/200 000 should rapidly (within 3 minutes) show if the drug has entered the subarachnoid space or a vessel directly.

No regional spinal anaesthesia technique is entirely predictable, and therefore success is dependent on meticulous monitoring and appropriate care of inadequate or excessive block.

Although the subarachnoid procedure is simpler, quicker and more reliable than the epidural, the latter is more flexible, with the possibility of extending the block and increasing its duration. From the original work of Dr Phillip Bromage, the dose of local anaesthetic required peridurally to reach a certain level was considered to be much less in the elderly, particularly those with arteriosclerosis or diabetes. More recently, this has been disputed and it does seem unclear. Certainly in the 60–90-year range there does not appear to be a need to decrease the dose of agent per segment. However, the required volume and concentration of drug injected (Table 5.2) do seem less in those over 60 compared with those under 60. Caudal epidural block shows no correlation between age and segmental spread.

With older patients one major difficulty is the flexion of the

---

*Subarachnoid bupivacaine + glucose 0.5 ml and 2 ml can extend over a saddle area and to T4 respectively—extradurally, approximately 0.75 ml is required to block each nerve segment.

**Table 5.2**
*Spinal analgesic drugs*

| Drug | Subarachnoid | Epidural |
|------|-------------|----------|
| Bupivacaine | 0.5% + 9.5% glucose<br>0.5% plain | 0.5% plain |
| Procaine | 5% | 2% |
| Lignocaine | 5% + 7.5% glucose | 1.5–2% |
| Etidocaine | | 1.0–1.5% |
| Prilocaine | 5% + 5% glucose | 3% (max. 600 mg) |

spine required for these techniques—the sitting position may be helpful but may be difficult to adopt. Distortion of the spine is also common, and getting the shoulders and hips perpendicular to the table in the lateral position is not always possible. A successful puncture will depend on a variety of techniques and the experience of the anaesthetist. A full understanding of the anatomy, the lateral approach and stepping along the bone can be invaluable. If a needle is passed between the posterior spinal processes towards an interspinal opening, contacts bone (*A*) and is then withdrawn and directed more cephalad where it contacts bone less deeply (*B*), then the opening is more caudal (*O*). Conversely, if on contacting bone (*X*), being withdrawn and reinserted more cephalad, it contacts bone more deeply (*Y*) then the space is more cephalad (*O*) (Fig. 5.6).

## Anaesthesia maintenance

If the induction of anaesthesia or block has been undertaken in an anteroom, moving to the operating theatre requires great care. Steps should be taken to maintain optimal respiratory status—ventilating the patient and/or administering oxygen in transit. Movement should be gentle and smooth so that there is no trauma or major vascular change due to postural mismanagement. Within the operating theatre it should be possible to control the heat of the room accurately because heat balance of the old is a major concern. For all but the most minor operations, this also requires either a heat exchanger or heated humidifier within the respiratory anaesthetic system and a warming mattress below the patient's body, together with

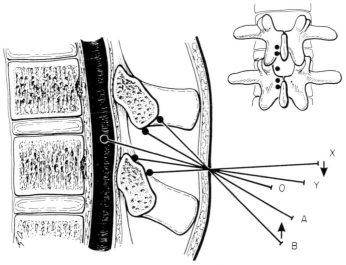

**Fig. 5.6** A sagittal section of the lumbar spine indicating the bony landmarks contacted by a needle directed to the subarachnoid space (see text).

temperature monitoring. To prevent body temperature loss a micro-atmosphere should be created by careful covering of the unoperated areas with appropriate material, and respiratory gases should be properly heated. Surgical irrigation and intravenous fluids should be at body temperature. Ripple-type mattresses are available for operating tables and are valuable for long procedures in avoiding excessive pressure in weight-bearing areas. A combined heated and ripple movement mattress through which x-ray is possible is uniquely satisfactory (Hawksley ripple heater).

For maintenance of anaesthesia, nitrous oxide, provided it is administered with sufficient oxygen, is emminently satisfactory because of its inherent safety and controllability. Every general anaesthetic reduces the FRC and this reduction is closely related to age. With the larger fall in FRC of an old patient, the relatively larger physiological shunt is further affected. Thus inspired oxygen must be relatively increased in the elderly and even more at high altitude. Augmenting anaesthesia with narcotics or volatile anaesthetic drugs should be relatively decreased. There is argument over whether narcotics or inhalation anaesthetics are the best, but a combination utilising the better qualities of both in minimal amounts would seem best, with doses varied in response to the individual's required change of depth of anaesthesia with differing intensity of surgical stimuli. With spontaneous ventilation, the maximum inspired concentration of halothane should rarely be over 1% in order to minimise cardiovascular and respiratory effects. With poor ventilation, blood pressure and heart rhythm, halothane must be removed and breathing assisted or controlled. Alternatively, enflurane up to 1% may be tried cautiously or small doses of narcotic used to maintain anaesthesia. When an operation requires relaxation, or progressive underventilation occurs (often beyond 40 minutes anaesthesia duration), controlled ventilation is indicated. Often controlled ventilation with nitrous oxide and little anaesthetic vapour and/or narcotic will provide adequate relaxation.

Specific relaxants must be employed in lower than usual doses (one-quarter to one-third, of adult dose) and rarely within 30 minutes of the end of a procedure. For long-term adjustments a nerve stimulator, with a 'train-of-four' mechanism, can be invaluable. Otherwise the clinical understanding of duration, wound 'tightness' and reduced ventilatory compliance are the only indications of increased need. Many surgeons require administration of antibiotics intravenously with the commencement of surgery; these are best diluted and administered slowly as they may cause convulsions. The aminoglycosides when given in large doses may, of course seriously, affect the relaxant duration.

## Artificial ventilation

When artificial ventilation is employed, much consideration must be given to the minute volume as this is often excessive and does not allow for the reduced carbon dioxide output of older patients. The serious effects on cerebral circulation of the reduced $Paco_2$ is a matter of conjecture and hypothesis (Fig. 5.7 and Fig. 5.8). A $Paco_2$ less than 25 mmHg (3.3 kPa) is also said to reduce cardiac output, increase peripheral resistance, and reduce flow in the coronary vessels (with consequent myocardial ischaemia or refactory arrhythmias). Each 10 mmHg (1.3 kPa) reduction in $Paco_2$ is also associated with a reduction of serum potassium by 0.5 mmol/l. Alkalaemia will

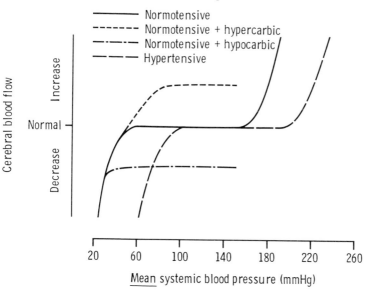

**Fig. 5.7** A diagrammatic indication of autoregulation of cerebral circulation in relation to mean systemic blood pressure, as affected by hypertension and different arterial carbon dioxide levels.

reduce oxygen tissue availability by shifting the oxygen – haemoglobin dissociation curve to the left. All of these changes are obviously more crucial in the aged. The Radford nomogram, or a simplification (70 ml/kg per min), can be applied together with expired carbon dioxide monitoring with a capnograph or, more rarely, intermittent $Paco_2$ measurements. Large tidal volumes are best avoided with old lung tuberculosis in order to reduce the risk of spreading infection or rupturing a bulla or emphysema. Spontaneous respiration may only restart at the preoperative $Paco_2$ level. With proper ventilation, safe light planes of anaesthesia, and drug antagonism when required, poor ventilation in recovery is a rare consequence.

## Extra attention

All anaesthetised elderly patients will benefit from the application of intermittent compression by a pump system on the legs during their immobile operative period. The position adopted for the operation requires careful adjustment to avoid

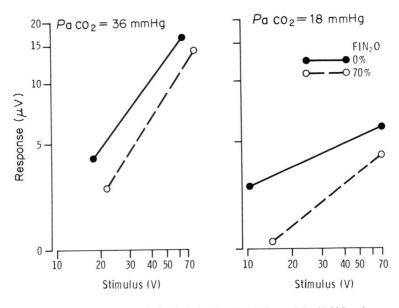

**Fig. 5.8** The response and stimuli relationship of evoked potentials with high and low $Pa_{CO_2}$ in people breathing oxygen or 70% nitrous oxide.

neurological, soft tissue or ligamentous damage, allowance being made for immobility of the various joints, which may be seriously damaged even by trying to adopt a physiological posture. No positioning should be grossly abnormal and padding should be freely used. In the case of a sedated or conscious patient undergoing local analgesia, great attention should be given to the comfort of the patient and this may entail quite unusual sitting or strangely supported positions which the patient can best tolerate.

Throughout these procedures the anaesthtist should explain to and support the patient, making sure that he or she understands that any painful experience will be dealt with. Because the patient may be restless, it is essential that the limbs be lightly restrained (not strapped down) so that sudden obstructive or disruptive movements are avoided. This may be accomplished by a belt across the knees and a bandage restraint of the wrists with the arms flexed. In the event of a patient feeling pain, surgery should be stopped while further analgesia is provided by *in situ* catheter injections, by epidural top-up, or by local infiltration by the surgeon. If it is apparent that the patient suffers from anxiety, general discomfort or disorientation, intravenous or inhalation sedation or hypnosis is called for. Inhalation agents are often preferable because of their inherent controllability, but hypotension, nausea and vomiting may be less with some of the newer intravenous drugs. At all times, drugs liable to be required and the instruments for airway management must be on hand. During maintenance of anaesthesia the other main requirement, apart from satisfactory anaesthesia and operating conditions, is the constant estimation of the homoeostasis of the patient.

## Transfusion

Because hypovolaemia is poorly tolerated in the elderly, it is necessary to estimate and measure blood loss in all but the most minor undertakings. When blood volumes were first estimated it was suggested that older patients coming for operations were commonly hypovolaemic, and thus liberal use of transfusion was advised. This view is now modified, and apart from recognising that there will be limited cardiac contractibility and vasodilation, the possibility of overload should also be borne in mind. Following the clinical signs of full peripheral veins and good perfusion, limb temperature maintenance, little systolic pressure reduction, together with routine direct arterial and central venous pressure measurement in any major undertaking should enable correct transfusion replacement.

When major changes in blood volume occur in a patient with poor or strained myocardium, the use of a Swan–Ganz catheter in the pulmonary artery may be necessary to measure left arterial pressure (LAP), but experience in its use shows it is not an easy undertaking. Because much of the blood now available is plasma reduced, there is particular concern about the correct mix of these units and other volume-replacing substances to ensure the viscosity is not raised. The dangers of increased viscosity are heightened in the elderly owing to the tendency for cardiac output, renal and cerebral blood flow to be reduced, together with a tendency to increased peripheral resistance. To provide the least ill-effect from transfusion to the elderly, it may also be necessary to use ultrafiltration routinely, to warm fluids to body temperature, and to add calcium gluconate and sodium bicarbonate judiciously. The use of multi-electrolyte solution to replace translocated fluid is permissible in the elderly provided the electrolyte corrections preoperatively have been within the acceptable ranges. If not, the necessary additions or subtractions made to a standard infusion of 6 ml/kg per hour will require special justification. When available, the urinary output is also monitored and 0.5–1 ml/kg per hour should be the aim. There are occasions when urgent blood sugar or potassium and acid-based analyses are indicated and these should be readily available in larger institutions.

## Electrocardiograms

Single-lead electrocardiography monitoring must be recognised as being severely limited in detecting both arrhythmias and ischaemic changes. The $V_1$ and $V_5$ leads would be ideal, respectively, but require five electrodes; thus use of a compromise $CM_5$ is now advised for the usual bipolar limb lead cardioscope. The right-arm lead is placed on the right shoulder (negative), the left-leg lead on the left anterior axillary line fifth interspace (positive), and the ground lead on the left shoulder. The lead selector will be on lead 111, and will indicate the grossest arrhythmias and sometimes major ischaemic changes to which older patients are prone. For arrhythmias, the gamut of therapeutic agents — atropine, lignocaine, verapamil and beta-blockers — need cautious use after ensuring correction of $Paco_2$, $Pao_2$ and hypovolaemia or hypotension.

Pacemakers are subject to interference by electromagnetic signals. Skeletal muscle myopotentials, due to shivering or suxamethonium fasciculation rarely interfere with pacing and the cardiogram in older patients. Diathermy, electrocautery, nerve stimulators, dental pulp testers, neurosurgical radio-frequency equipment or any electric motor does interfere. Although the newer pacemakers are shielded and filtered to reduce malfunction, monitoring is essential because of these possibilities. Ground electrodes and devices should be away from the pacemaker and short leads will give less signal; short bursts of cautery, preferably with bipolar forceps, may be permissible.

## Hypotensive techniques

It would rarely appear to be wise to employ a deliberate hypotensive technique in the elderly as the conditions for its use are that it adds no extra danger and is essential for the particular operation. The limits of safety with arteriosclerosis, hypertension or reduced cerebral blood flow (all of which may be undiagnosed in an old patient) have not been defined. Also there are very few operations which cannot be accomplished without severe hypotension being produced. It is best therefore applied only by those most proficient in the techniques.

### Further reading

*Induction*
Christensen J.H. *et al.* (1981). Influence of age and sex on the pharmacokinetics of thiopentone. *Brit. J. Anaesth*; **53**:1189.
Christensen J.H. *et al.* (1983). Thiopentone sensitivity in young and elderly women. *Brit. J. Anaesth*; **55**:33.
Cummings M.F. *et al.* (1983). The effect of suxamethonium and d-tubocurarine on the pressor and plasma catecholamine responses to tracheal intubation. *Anaesth. Int. Care*; **11**:103.
Cummings M.F. *et al.* (1983). Effects of pancuronium and alcuronium on the changes in arterial pressure and plasma catecholamine concentration during tracheal intubation. *Brit. J. Anaesth*; **55**:619.
Dahlgren N., Messeter K. (1981). Treatment of stress response to laryngoscopy and intubation with fentanyl. *Anaesth*; **36**:1022.
Dundee J.W., Hassard T.H. (1983). The influence of haemoglobin and plasma urea levels on the induction dose of thiopentone. *Anaesth*; **38**:26.
Gamble J.A. *et al.* (1981). Evaluation of midazolam as an intravenous induction agent. *Anaesth*; **36**:868.
Gold M.I. *et al.* (1981). Arterial oxygen after 30 seconds $O_2$ breathing. *Anesth. Analg*; **6**:313.
Hoffman P. *et al.* (1980). Intravenous short narcosis in geriatric patients. *Acta Anaesthesiol. Belg*; **31**:249.
Jung D. *et al.* (1982). Thiopental disposition as a function of age in female patients undergoing surgery. *Anesthesiol*; **56**:263.
Kofman A.F. *et al.* (1975). Awake endotracheal intubation — a review of 267 cases. *Anesth. Analg*; **54**:323.
Lorhan P.H. (1971). Clinical appraisal of the use of ketamine hydrochloride in the aged. *Anesth. Analg*; **50**:323.
Muravchick S. (1984). Effect of age and premed on thiopental sleep dose. *Anesthesiol*; **61**:333.
Pakkanen A., Kanto J. (1982). Midazolam compared with thiopentone as an induction agent. *Acta Anaesthesiol. Scand*; **26**(2):143.
Pedersen P. (1971). Blind nasotracheal intubation review. *Acta Anaesthesiol. Scand*; **15**:107.
Pontoppidan H., Beecher H.K. (1960). Progressive loss of protective reflexes in the airway with advancing age. *J. Am. Med. Assoc*; **174**:2209.
Stovner J. *et al.* (1972). Suxamethonium hyperkalaemia with different induction agents. *Acta Anaesthesiol. Scand*; **16**(1):46.

*Regional anaesthesia*
Andersen S., Cold G.E. (1981). Dose response studies in elderly patients subjected to epidural analgesia. *Acta Anaesthesiol. Scand*; **25**(3):279.
Austin T.R. (1980). Low dose ketamine and diazepam during spinal analgesia. *Anaesth*; **35**:391.

Backer C.L. *et al.* (1979). Myocardial reinfarction following local anaesthesia. *Anesthesiol*; **51**(Suppl.):S61.

Bergenwald L. *et al.* (1981). Cardiovascular response to spinal anaesthesia in elderly men: effects of head-up tilt and dihydroergotamine administration. *Clin. Physiol*; **1**(5):453.

Bromage P.R. (1969). Ageing and epidural dose requirement. *Brit. J. Anaesth*; **41**:1016.

Cameron A.E. *et al.* (1981). Spinal analgesia using bupivacaine 0.5% plain — variations in the extent of the block with patient age. *Anaesth*; **36**:318.

Dagnino J., Prys-Roberts C. (1984). Studies of anaesthesia in relation to hypertension: cardiovascular responses to extradural blockade of treated and untreated hypertensive patients. *Brit. J. Anaesth*; **56**:1065.

Dohi S. *et al.* (1979). Age related changes in blood pressure and duration of motor block in spinal anaesthesia. *Anesthesiol*; **50**:319.

Freund P.R. *et al.* (1984). Caudal anesthesia with lidocaine and bupivacaine plasma local anesthetic concentration and extent of spread in old and young patients. *Anesth. Analg*; **63**:1017.

Howard C.B. *et al.* (1983). Femoral neck surgery using a local anaesthetic technique. *Anaesth*; **38**:993.

Marley J.E., Ward S. (1980). Chlormethiazole as sleep cover for the elderly. Intravenous infusion during local analgesia. *Anaesth*; **35**(4):386.

Mulroy M.F. *et al.* (1977). Age, chronic obstructive pulmonary disease and INOVAR induced ventilatory depression during regional anaesthesia. *Anesth. Analg*; **56**:826.

Park W.Y. *et al.* (1975). Effects of patient age, pH of cerebrospinal fluid and vasopressors on the onset and duration of spinal anaesthesia. *Anesth. Analg*; **54**:455.

Park W.Y. *et al.* (1982). Age and epidural dose response in adult men. *Anesthesiol*; **56**:318.

Pearce C. (1974). The respiratory effects of diazepam supplementation of spinal anaesthesia in elderly males. *Brit. J. Anaesth*; **46**(6):439.

Pitkanen M., Haapaniemi L., Tuominen M., Rosenburg P.H. (1984). Influence of age on spinal anaesthesia with isobaric 0.5% bupivacaine. *Brit. J. Anaesth*; **56**(3):279.

Rosenberg P.H., Saramies L., Alila A. (1984). Lumbar epidural anaesthesia with bupivacaine in old patients: effect of speed and duration of injection. *Acta Anaesthesiol. Scand*; **25**(3):270.

Sharrock N.E. (1978). Epidural anaesthetic dose responses in patients 20 to 80 years old. *Anesthesiol*; **49**:425.

Sharrock N.E. *et al.* (1984). Segmental levels of anaesthesia following the extradural injection of 0.75% bupivacaine at different lumbar spaces in elderly patients. *Brit. J. Anaesth*; **56**:285.

### Maintenance

Alroy G. *et al.* (1966). Respiratory studies associated with general anaesthesia and controlled ventilation in elderly patients. *Acta Anaesthesiol. Scand*; **23**(Suppl. B):203.

Dinnick O.P. (1980). *In Somno Securitas*—a sermon in safety. *Scott. Soc. Anaesth. Newsletter*; **21**:17.

Editorial (1981). Effects of ventilation on circulation. *Brit. Med. J*; **1**:283.

Hardesty W.H. *et al.* (1960). Studies of carotid artery flow in man. *New Engl. J. Med*; **263**:944.

Marshall B.E., Wyche M.Q. (1972). Hypoxaemia during and after anaesthesia. *Anesthesiol*; **37**:178.

Prys-Roberts C., Kelman G.R. (1967). The influence of drugs used in neuroleptanalgesia on cardiovascular and respiratory function. *Brit. J. Anaesth*; **39**:134.

Prys-Roberts C. *et al.* (1972). Studies of anaesthesia in relation to hypertension: IV. The effects of artificial ventilation on the circulation and pulmonary gas exchanges. *Brit. J. Anaesth*; **44**:335.

Yamaguichi F. *et al.* (1979). Normal human ageing and cerebral vasoconstrictive responses to hypocapnia. *J. Neurol. Sci*; **44**:87.

# CHAPTER 6

# The postoperative period

## Early recovery

Modern anaesthetists accept that the postoperative period is a major concern of theirs, as well as of the surgeons. The preparation and anaesthetic management of the patient should be undertaken with the intent of keeping the postoperative period as free of problems as is possible. However, even the greatest care and attention given to assessment and management of an anaesthetic can be wasted if the postoperative period is mismanaged. The end of any anaesthetic is indefinable, and some of the contents of this chapter would usually be included in a description of the anaesthetic itself. This arrangement of subjects for postanaesthetic concern recognises the continuum of care which is so essential.

### Neuromuscular block

Except in patients who are to be continuously artificially ventilated, it is usual to antidote the non-depolarising relaxant's effect by the routine administration of anticholinesterase drug. This is only permissible if there is evidence of some return of neuromuscular transmission. To minimise the effect of the anticholinesterase agent on the heart, it is essential that controlled or assisted ventilation is maintained and the $Paco_2$ is as near normal as possible during reversal. The routine of antidote administration after the use of a relaxant with the expectation of a return of immediate full muscular power required to overcome any ventilation problem, is not justifiable in many elderly patients. Anticholinergic drugs are needed to reduce the side-effects of the antidote, but whether it is preferable to use the two drugs in combination or sequentially is undecided. Because the unwanted 'muscarinic' effects (especially those on the heart) occur more frequently in the elderly for up to 90 minutes after use of the antidote, it is suggested that pyridostigmine with glycopyrronium is preferable.

Anticholinergic drug effects in the elderly will be less apparent, but their use for antisecretory or antiperistaltic activity requires prior injection—with a period of 3 minutes allowed for full effect and a further 12 minutes for observing the total response to an anticholinesterase drug. To ensure that this happens under the observation of the anaesthetist, it may be wise to administer the drugs during closure of the deeper layers of the wound so that good spontaneous ventilation can be present by the end of the operation. This is more acceptable in the elderly and aged because their objection to the *in situ* tube is clearly less marked, and any awareness of the prolonged intubation can be obtunded by the correct use of anaesthetics or narcotics. Other antidotes of recognised use after anaesthesia, such as physostigmine, doxapram and naloxone, should rarely be required, but may well be more frequently indicated for older patients than for the young.

*Extubation*

Transfer from the operating theatre to the recovery room may be safer with retention of an endotracheal tube in a considerable number of old patients. The indications for delayed extubation include delay in fully reflexive consciousness, a modicum of residual ventilatory decrease, the possibility of aspiration combined with diminished protective reflexes in the airway, any minor degree of hypoxia, or when a position other than the lateral is needed. All of these indications readily apply to the old, so that a major proportion of recovering patients should have an endotracheal tube in place. In the case of a 'wet' chest problem, it is very beneficial to have assisted coughing—to suction the end of an *in situ* endotracheal tube intermittently during recovery so that as much intralung débris as possible is removed at this critical period.

*Oxygenation*

Diffusion hypoxia may be more serious and prolonged in the elderly. The perioperative mismatch of ventilation to perfusion in the lungs increases with age, and is marked after major operations. Therefore postoperative routine oxygen administration should continue for as long as tolerable, whatever the

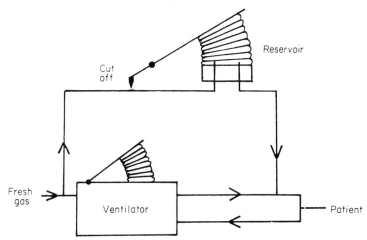

**Fig. 6.1** A diagrammatic representation of a mandatory minute volume circuit. (Note that directional valves are omitted.)

previous anaesthetic technique. The concentration administered has to be limited in hypercapnic patients, but a rise of 5–10% in inspired oxygen is usually sufficient. In the presence of shivering (not common in the elderly), the oxygen uptake does rise dramatically two- or threefold. This oxygen demand is greatest in the rapidly awakened, pain-racked very old patient who has had major blood loss. The increase of ventilation and cardiac output to satisfy the demand is then not readily produced. Fifteen minutes after an anaesthetic the $Pao_2$ can approximate

$$80 - \frac{\text{age}}{4} \text{ mmHg}$$

or less, with impaired reserves in respiratory dynamics which we do not often assess preoperatively. The $Paco_2$ is raised in half the elderly postoperative patients but not as frequently in the very old. Conversely, the latter are more likely to have a low $Paco_2$. Patients who have had major operations and are undergoing the progressive redistribution and elimination of the drug they have been given, and who have metabolic changes arising from the anaesthetic and operation, may benefit from a gradual reinstitution of their own breathing patterns and volumes. This can best be achieved by mandatory minute volume administration of oxygen-enriched air (Fig. 6.1). A monitored preselected minute volume of fresh gas, from which the patient breathes as much as he or she is able, is provided, with the remainder being delivered via a ventilator. If the reservoir bag fills, its inlet is occluded and the gas diverts to a minute volume-dividing ventilator which delivers a controlled tidal volume to the patient. All fresh gases therefore enter the patient's lungs as a result of the patient's efforts or the action of the ventilator.

### Cardiovascular state

After ventilation, the second concern is the haemodynamic state of the patient which can be assessed crudely by means of a continuous measurement of urinary output. Routine use of a catheter in the bladder always carries with it a danger of introducing infection, but with careful sterile precautions and closed drainage, urine should be bacteria free for 5–7 days. This and other monitoring is relied upon while recognising that 3–4 hours are required for stabilisation of the vital systems, provided there are no acute changes. Thus the period of equalisation of central and peripheral temperatures coincides with that of haemodynamic instability—hence the equating of the generalised satisfactory perfusion with a return to the preoperative level of the temperature of the great toe. A structured clinical assessment combined in a scoring system may help provide a better idea of a patient's recovery (see Appendix E5). A postoperative scoring system may be especially helpful for the more junior nurse who does not have sufficient clinical experience to assess the elderly patient properly. The ECG, intravascular pressures, blood gas analysis or other means of monitoring must be applied when indicated. A balance of the fluid input and output, with the further replacement of translocated fluids or other extravascular losses, should be routine and take full account of the previous carefully noted intraoperative administrations and losses. When urinary output is not adequate (due to prerenal causes) after more than adequate correction of hypovolaemia, intravenous frusemide can be administered early as a prophylactic measure to avoid renal shutdown. Mannitol infusion is considered more scientific by some renal physicians.

### Inappropriate secretion of antidiuretic hormone (ADH)

The antidiuretic hormone (arginine vasopressin of the

posterior pituitary gland) is released by severe haemodynamic changes. Contrary to earlier views, increased anaesthesia or narcotic doses suppress the release of ADH. On occasion, stress response to intense stimulation, hypovolaemia, hypotension, hypoxia, hypercarbia, changed plasma osmotic pressure or some drugs produce 'inappropriate' amounts of ADH. This is most common in elderly patients and is indicated by low serum osmolality (<235 osmol/l), hyponatraemia, and excretion of hypertonic urine occurring up to a week after an operation. The condition presents with restlessness progressing to coma from a dilutional or direct ADH effect on the brain cells. Drastic fluid restriction, cautious sodium administration and attention to other physiological derangements is required.

## Temperature

Temperature control may require quite prolonged attention and it must be realised that hypothermia is a frequent occurrence in the modern operating room environment. In one set of circumstances, 60% of patients on arrival in the recovery room had a temperature of less than 36°C, and 1 in 10 of less than 35°C (up to 20% of the patients were actually shivering). This situation could be prevented if the temperature of operating theatres were not set for the comfort of surgeons and other staff. Because of poor heat balance, old patients will generally be found to have a lower temperature throughout their time in the recovery room (Fig. 6.2); this occurs after regional local analgesia as much as after a general anaesthetic.

The temperature should be recorded, and rewarming used for every patient requiring it—recognising the hypothermic effect on drug elimination and the rather prolonged course of core-to-peripheral temperature equalisation. Reduction of temperature fall has been shown to diminish proteolysis and nitrogen excretion dramatically.

## Other care

Any diabetic subject, even although fully conscious, should have an early blood sugar estimation. If a patient experiences severe pain, a chosen analgesic should be administered incrementally intravenously, but only after attention for any

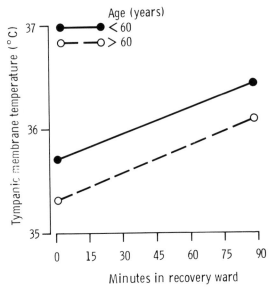

**Fig. 6.2** The temperature recordings of old and young patients in the first 90 minutes postoperatively.

shock or hypoxia. If there is iatrogenic confusion immediately postoperatively, this can often be aborted by incremental intravenous physostigmine (0.5 mg every 5 minutes). Physostigmine acts in 3 minutes and lasts 40–60 minutes. It reduces respiratory rate depression and somnolence without antidoting any analgesia present. It has been shown to counter overdose of morphine, diazepam, fentanyl, ketamine and tricyclic antidepressants. The most common causes of slow recovery of consciousness are drugs, hypothermia, hypoglycaemia and myxoedema.

For patients chronically mentally disturbed, judicious use of droperidol or chlorpromazine may be helpful. The vasodilatory property of these drugs must be allowed for, together with their potentiation of sedatives and narcotics. Their sparing use is advocated because they may produce symptoms associated with extrapyramidal lesions, for example oculogyric crisis, hypertonia with respiratory elements, and agitation. The limited duration of action of neostigmine and naloxone may well require their repeated postoperative injection if muscle relaxation or respiratory depression becomes apparent again. In some patients a semirecumbent position will be appreciated whenever it is feasible. Although this has little effect on the $Pao_2$, the ventilatory 'appropriateness' does seem enhanced with consequent reduced dyspnoea.

A mundane consideration is the fixation of a nasogastric tube. This requires mention because too frequently it is extremely uncomfortable for the patient or it may not be retained in a patient when it is essential, for example with oesophageal reconstruction or distal placement after complex bowel bypass procedures (Fig. 6.3). In the latter instances, strong adhesive tape reinforced with skin adhesives will be found invaluable. For the immobile patient during recovery, continuation of the leg pumping, particularly in those most at risk of pulmonary embolism, should be undertaken until active leg movements are carried out. A particular problem is the management of a Helmstein bladder dilatation. This entails 7–8 hours of continuous epidural block for the abolition of the discomfort of the distended bladder. In some cases this may need supplementary sedative or a continuous anaesthetic infusion. Patients with residual local anaesthetic blocks must be protected from postural damage or heater burns, as must all those who are generally unresponsive. Also, postural changes must not be excessive for fear of producing severe hypotension.

Postoperative vomiting is less common in the elderly (approximately 18%), and other than an anaesthetic cause must be sought more often. Other 'minor' sequelae, for example headache, dizziness, sore throat and suxamethonium muscle pains, are all reported less often in older patients. Local anaesthetic injected into operation wounds routinely will cause a slower, calmer return to consciousness after general anaesthesia. Pain diminished in this way also facilitates the use of narcotic antidotes without the seesaw changes of discomfort or depression. When the simpler causes of hypertension (hypercapnia, shivering, hypoxia and pain) have been managed, it is uncommon to see persistent postoperative hypertension. Such essential hypertension postoperatively can be associated with tachycardia, pulmonary oedema or myocardial ischaemia. A diastolic pressure greater than 120 mmHg should therefore be treated with 5 mg of hydrallazine intravenously (repeated if necessary at 5-minute intervals). When there is a sustained tachycardia as well, it should be treated with intravenous labetalol (2–5 mg/h).

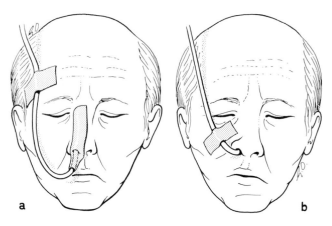

a                                                       b

**Fig. 6.3** A method of fixation of a nasogastric tube which is efficient and comfortable (a) compared with an uncomfortable attachment (b).

## Remote recovery

### *Pain relief*

The anaesthetist's involvement in ward care postoperatively is too often limited. This may be due to a lack of available time but too frequently is because of historical non-involvement in an area where he or she may contribute much to the total recovery of patients. This applies especially to pain control which requires that all the nursing and medical staff looking after a patient postoperatively understand the very variable needs of different patients after different operations and ensure that these needs are dealt with effectively and efficiently at all times. Once a ward becomes 'pain conscious', the success rate of their interventions will be markedly increased. Whatever method is employed, the first concern must be that it does not represent an added danger. In this respect, the preoperative education of patients about the availability of pain relief and its proper administration can reduce anxiety and will inevitably reduce drug needs. Cooperation and acceptance of some discomforts will be dependent on the personality of the patient. Whereas in younger age groups nervous types have been proven to require more analgesia postoperatively, in the aged the overall need appears to be diminished as the amount of anxiety is reduced.

Relief of pain immediately postoperatively seems most vital in regard to future requirements of analgesia—that is, if a patient does not initially experience severe pain, then the total requirement of analgesic over the following days is reduced. Continuous analgesic conduction block would be ideal, but in a majority of operations it is not a practical alternative to narcotics. It is said that abdominal and thoracic operations inflict the most postoperative pain, but assessment of pain quantity is exceedingly difficult, and on occasions it would appear that some bone surgery can produce severe pain.

When narcotics are used, it must be clearly understood that their depressant effect on the cardiovascular and respiratory systems and the bowel, together with urinary retention and nausea, make their use less than totally satisfactory. In principle, the longest acting narcotics may seem the most rational, for example methadone or buprenorphine, but if there is a changing requirement and side-effects are to be avoided or reduced to a minimum, short-acting drugs given continuously may be more rational. This is especially so in the very sick and the elderly.

Continuous intravenous, intramuscular or subcutaneous administration with a pump-driven syringe may be the most suitable methods of administering drugs, provided the requirement is assessed at frequent intervals, with adjustments of rate made as necessary (see Fig. 11.1). The automated self-administration demand system is less suitable for the aged because of its complexity and the cooperation required on behalf of the patient for its correct use. The principle of patients withstanding a minimal amount of discomfort and not being made completely pain free would seem preferable because in this way serious complications will not be masked and the dangers are considerably reduced. When a patient has to undergo painful procedures, such as physiotherapy and mobilisation, there will clearly be an exacerbation of pain and this may be best dealt with by an additional injection or the administration of Entonox. It is usual for pain to become less on the second or third day postoperatively, and if this is not so a complication should be suspected and sought for. Resistance to analgesia is also evident in those who are hyperanxious, and in this case a pure tranquilliser may be of considerable benefit in producing sedation which will fortify recuperation. Once the pain is less severe, many alternative non-parenteral forms of analgesia are available and should be more widely used. When some of the later pain is due to inflammatory reaction, a non-steroidal anti-inflammatory drug may be quite effective.

Some analgesics may be administered by the sublingual or rectal route when indicated and in this instance long action is preferable. The use of a transcutaneous electrical nerve stimulator is an innocuous, useful supplementary method for some patients when the pain is not severe or in conjunction with other methods. The use of extradural and intrathecal narcotics must at present be considered experimental and their full assessment is awaited.

### Respiratory care

Preoperative education concerning the need for regular deep breathing and coughing as required after an operation is essential. The patient's usual inclination and intent is to avoid any strain upon the operative wound in the belief that this would be detrimental to recovery or to the surgical handicraft. Reinforcement of encouragement to breathe deeply must be given by the nursing and physiotherapy staff.

It must be recognised that the reflexes which protect the airway are progressively less efficient with ageing. The provision of adequate pain relief is an important factor in permitting the full expansion of the lungs, provided that the drugs administered are not also causing severe respiratory depression or diminishing muscular power, as with epidural block. Awareness of the fact that a pneumothorax may be created by an operative or anaesthetic mishap is important. If there is proper humidification of administered gases during the anaesthetic, it is frequently found that the $Pao_2$ will be at a higher level for 1–5 days and there will be a decreased incidence of cough, sputum or chest signs.

The use of stimulants (such as doxapram) may be indicated postoperatively in an attempt to ensure that there are no atelectatic areas produced within the lungs through extended sedation. Very careful counting of the respiratory rate is valuable as a sign of lung complications. If unaffected by drugs, the normal range of respiratory rate is 16–25 breaths/min, and any patient with a higher rate should have extra careful respiratory assessment. Tachypnoea is fairly specific with acute postoperative respiratory dysfunction and in one study affected patients had a mean rate of 29.7/minute. Whenever it appears that there is atelectasis, active treatment by physiotherapy, suction within the pharynx or trachea, and intermittent positive pressure ventilation of humidified gas and drugs can be curative. Antibiotics are required when there are special lung complications, but their routine prophylactic use in other than chest surgery has not been proved to be helpful. A minitracheotomy, suction through a fibre-optic bronchoscope or a conventional tracheostomy should be used at an early rather than late stage. Minitracheotomy requires the least expertise.

*Cardiovascular care*

Cardiovascular support is as for younger patients, except that it should be very prompt and there must be constant awareness of the high incidence of collapse if remedial action is insufficient. Postoperative failure is usually associated with previous disease of the heart, particularly myocardial infarction, and possibly with amyloidosis of the aged. A thyrotoxic state or anaemia can be a precipitating factor which must be eliminated. Special attention must be given to the required potassium supplementation when diuretics are employed and the fact that the efficient action of frusemide may precipitate retention of urine in older men. Aminophylline adminstered intravenously can have a valuable inotropic effect. The need for paracentesis, especially of the pleura, may be evident and should always be remembered. Digitalis is much used if there is auricular fibrillation, which is the most common arrhythmia. However, if the auricular fibrillation is slow, there would appear to be no need to treat it, only when it is fast and uncontrollable should paediatric doses of digitalis be employed. The addition of propranolol may be helpful, particularly in hypertensive patients. The hypertensive patient who cannot take the necessary antihypertensive or antianginal drugs normally required by the oral route should be kept in intensive care for intravenous infusion of labetalol or atenolol.

*Deep vein thrombosis (DVT)*

This is the third condition for which preoperative education is of great value. Exercising of leg muscles frequently and vigorously, with minimal bed rest, will be most readily acceptable and the discomfort involved may be tolerated more when an explanation is given to patients of how it will assist rehabilitation.

Because sophisticated diagnostic tests are proposed but difficult to undertake, it is important to remember the clinical signs of thrombosis or embolism. Major vein involvement may be suggested by classic leg pains, abdominal discomfort, ventral or iliac fossae, as well as by buttock or sciatic pain or deep pelvic, rectum or bladder discomfort.

Any atypical pneumonia not responding to antibiotics, especially with haemoptysis, suggests lung embolism. The symptoms of multiple pulmonary embolism can be minor, for example fever, faints, tachycardia or dry cough. The classic triad of dyspnoea, haemoptysis and pleural pain occurs in only one-third of older affected patients. Signs of pulmonary embolism are not clear cut, but indicative ones are a DVT, bronchospasm, pleural rub, chest x-ray wedge opacity or pleural effusion. With DVT prophylaxis, one must be aware of the fact that warfarin produces a greater effect on the coagulation of an old patient compared with that of a young patient, at the same blood level of the drug.

*Other care*

The ward environment may on occasion be too cold, particularly when there is excessive exposure for medical attention, in nursing or drip management for example. Devices such as high air-flow beds or water mattresses may particularly affect the heat balance of the patient. The devices are usually employed only for those with a debilitated state and pressure necrosis—that is, those who would be most vulnerable to hypothermia.

Bowel ileus from operative handling or repair will occur more commonly because of the relative dysautonomia of older patients. An early application of a transcutaneous nerve stimulator to the abdominal wall may produce activation before it becomes resistant; this is an innocuous technique.

There have been few controlled studies of nutritional support in elderly patients postoperatively. It is logical to group patients and to aim to reduce the morbidity and rehabilitation time of the thinnest by supplementary feeding because their food intake is usually consistently low. This has been done most simply by overnight nasogastric tube feeding (see Chapter 8).

If intentional or accidental lumbar puncture leads to prolonged and severe headache owing to cerebrospinal fluid leakage, an epidural blood patch should be used because the unsupported brain may give rise to catastrophic consequences, for example subarachnoid haemorrhage.

### Mental changes

There is a strong reluctance by some anaesthetists to accept that anaesthesia itself can be a major factor in the mental deterioration that geriatricians and psychiatrists have sometimes observed postoperatively. This view stems, in recent times, from two classic papers often referred to. In 1955 an Oxford physician presented patients whom he believed had undergone sudden, acute deterioration of their mental state after having an operation with anaesthesia. He attributed this to hypoxia, starvation or drug effects. This led to a study, reported in 1961, by anaesthetists concerning a follow-up of all old patients anaesthetised in the same city for 1 year and comparing their mental state to that which had been apparent preoperatively. In essence this work disputes the original idea that operations with anaesthesia are detrimental to mental function in old patients. Such contrary views are similar to those which surround possible psychic trauma in children undergoing operations with anaesthesia. It would appear that in either childhood or old age any hospital admission or illness, which may involve surgery or anaesthesia, is liable to cause instability of the mental state of patients; this is usually of limited duration provided there has not been a major mental insult to those subjects who are at special risk. Also, those who are progressively deteriorating mentally will continue their progression at no greater rate unless they are mismanaged. Others, it must be noted, may improve mentally after a successful operation.

The evidence of detailed psychological studies and EEG recordings is that there are postanaesthetic changes which are liable to be more marked in the older patient but are not consistent. Lesser changes of mental capacity, such as alteration of memory and orientation, slurring speech and change in the kinds and degree of emotions, may only be noticeable to close friends and relatives. Electroencephalographs suggest subacute hypoxia, and 1 in 10 patients will show persistent changes—mostly patients with ventilation problems or myocardial infarction, and most commonly those over 80 years of age, undergoing operations lasting longer than 4 hours, or with considerable loss of blood (>1200 ml).

If psychometric testing is undertaken after an operation on a patient in hospital, there will be found to be a minor decrease in reaction times, finer movements and objective recognition. This is at a maximum 4–5 days postoperatively but may last up to 3 weeks. Along with the bed rest and surgery involved, the other causes could include starvation, sleep deprivation or the anaesthetic. In some patients there is quite a serious inferior test performance, particularly in the aged where one more frequently encounters the need for extensive surgery. Nevertheless, in comparable groups the difference between major and minor surgery is not obvious. An inferior performance includes the requirement to organise thought as well as the retention of fact. In some, a difficulty with vision is also experienced. All these deficits appeared to improve with time. A comparison with patients merely moved from one institution to another, rather than from home to a hospital, did not show any clear difference. Therefore the environmental change may not be very important. Whenever complications arise postoperatively, as shown by rising temperature or multiple drug use, there is, as expected, a tendency for poorer performance of tests. Psychiatrists accept that the tests used are of a type which are sensitive to damage at the cerebral cortex. In special studies, executive powers were unimpaired but perception or conceptional organisation of new material was affected. In psychiatric terms the condition is similar to that of an acute exogenous psychosis as would be apparent with, for example, LSD, alcohol, opium, hashish or amphetamines. There are often abreactive effects of forgotten experiences of an unpleasant nature and it is not improbable that an anaesthetic could act in the same way. This confused state may last up to 3 weeks.

It therefore seems we should accept that after surgery with anaesthesia the elderly may have mental disturbance of a slight degree. This generally takes the form of disorganisation of thought caused by many of the perioperative happenings, including the anaesthetic effect on the cerebral cortex. Children deeply disturbed mentally by hospital treatment are more prone to adolescent behavioural problems, and the postoperative confusion of elderly patients is four times as common in those who later become demented—whether these are inherent or cause-and-effect relationships is unproven. Regardless of this lack of proof, our aim must be to have undisturbed children and unconfused elders. This we can assist if we understand their feelings, provide stimulation, and explain to them repeatedly the details of their condition and its management as well as perfecting our anaesthetic care.

**Further reading**

*Immediate*

Bay J. *et al.* (1968). Factors influencing arterial $Po_2$ during recovery from anaesthesia. *Brit. J. Anaesth*; **40**:398.

Dentoch C. *et al.* (1966). Post operative hyponatraemia with inappropriate release of antidiuretic hormone. *Anesthesiol*; **27**:250.

Erikson S. *et al.* (1978). Effects on muscarinic receptors of various agents in reversal of neuromuscular blockade. *Acta Anaesthesiol. Scand*; **22**:447.

Fairley H.B. *et al.* (1968). The avoidance of post operative hypoxaemia: an assessment of three techniques for use during anaesthesia. *Can. Anaesth. Soc. J*; **15**:152.

Glissen S.M. *et al.* (1978). Amitriptyline therapy increases electrocardiographic changes during reversal of neuromuscular blockade. *Anesth. Analg*; **57**:77.

Hill G.E. *et al.* (1977). Physostigmine reversal of post operative somnolence. *Can. Anaesth. Soc. J*; **24**:707.

Kitamura H. *et al.* (1972). Post-operative hypoxaemia: the contribution of age to the maldistribution of ventilation. *Anesthesiol*; **36**:244.

Marshall B.E., Miller R.A. (1965). Some factors influencing post-operative hypoxaemia. *Anaesth*; **20**:408.

Morioka T. *et al.* (1980). Problems in neurosurgical operations on elderly patients from the viewpoint of anaesthesiology. *Neurol., Med. Chir*; **20**(7):713.

Muravchick D.H. *et al.* (1979). Glycopyrrolate and cardiac disrhythmias in geriatric patients after reversal of neuromuscular blockade. *Can. Anaesth. Soc. J*; **26**:22.

Nunn J.F. (1965). The influence of age and other factors on hypoxaemia in the post operative period. *Lancet*; **ii**:466.

Owens W.D. *et al.* (1978). Cardiac dysrhythmia following reversal of neuromuscular blocking agents in geriatric patients. *Anesth. Analg*; **57**:186.

Page M.M.B., Watkins J.B. (1981). Cardiorespiratory arrest and diabetic autonomic neuropathy. *Lancet*; **i**:14.

Roseberg B., Wulff K. (1981). Hemodynamics following normovolemic hemodilution in elderly patients. *Acta Anaesthesiol. Scand*; **25**(5):402.

Sevmmarken C. *et al.* (1984). Partial curarization in the post operative period. *Acta Anaesthesiol. Scand*; **28**:260.

Smith D.S. *et al.* (1979). Prolonged sedation in the elderly after intraoperative atropine administration. *Anesthesiol*; **51**:348.

Summers W.K., Reich T.C. (1979). Delirium after cataract surgery. *Am. J. Psych*; **136**:386.

Vaughan M.S. *et al.* (1981). Post operative hypothermia in adults: relationship of age, anesthesia and shivering to rewarming. *Anesth. Analg*; **60**(10):746.

Wishart H.Y. *et al.* (1977). A comparison of the effect of three anaesthetic techniques on post-operative arterial oxygenation in the elderly. *Brit. J. Anaesth*; **49**(12):1259.

*Remote*

Bedford P.D. (1955). Adverse cerebral effects of anaesthesia on old people. *Lancet*; **ii**:299.

Bellville J.W. *et al.* (1971). Age and pain relief. *J. Am. Med. Assoc*; **217**:1841.

Blundell E. (1967). A psychological study of the effect of surgery in 86 elderly patients. *Brit. J. Soc. Clin. Psych*; **6**:297.

Carli F. *et al.* (1982). Investigation of the relationship between heat loss and nitrogen excretion in the elderly patients undergoing major abdominal surgery under general anaesthetic. *Brit. J. Anaesth*; **54**:1023.

Ecrola M. *et al.* (1981). Fatal brain lesion following spinal anaesthesia. *Acta Anaesth. Scand*; **25**:115.

Edelman J.D., Wingard D.W. (1980). Subdural haematomas after lumbar dural puncture. *Anesthesiol*; **52**:166.

Edwards H. *et al.* (1981). Post-operative deterioration in psychomotor function. *J. Am. Med. Assoc*; **245**:1342.

Forrest W.H. *et al.* (1973). Dextramphetamine with morphine for the treatment of post operative pain. *New Engl. J. Med*; **296**:712.

Fridnowski R.J. (1969). The electro-encephalogram in older patients following prolonged surgery. *Anesth. Analg*; **48**:297.

Gredinsky C. (1974). Post-operative pulmonary complications in the geriatric age group. *J. Am. Geriatr. Soc*; **22**:208.

Kaiko R.F. (1980). Age and morphine analgesia in cancer patients with post operative pain. *Clin. Pharm. Ther*; **28**:823.

Matthews H.R., Hopkinson R.B. (1984). Treatment of sputum retention by mini tracheotomy. *Brit. J. Surg*; **71**:147.

Mauney F.M. *et al.* (1970). Post operative myocardial infarction. *Ann. Surg*; **172**:497.

Millar G.A.H. (1977). The management of acute pulmonary embolism. *Brit. J. Hosp. Med*; **18**:26.

Millar H.R. (1981). Psychiatric morbidity in elderly surgical patients. *Brit. J. Psych*; **138**:17.

Newrick P., Read D. (1977). Subdural haematoma as a complication of spinal anaesthesia. *Brit. Med. J*; **285**:845.

Renck H. (1969). The elderly patient after anaesthesia and surgery. *Acta Anaesthesiol. Scand*; (P Suppl.) **34**:1.

Rose E.A., King J.C. (1978). Post-operative fatigue. *Surg. Obstet. Gynaecol*; **147**:97.

Rudehill A. *et al.* (1983). Subdural haematoma: a rare but life-threatening complication after spinal anaesthesia. *Acta Anaesthesiol. Scand*; **27**(5): DL376.

Rüs J. *et al.* (1983). Immediate and long term mental recovery from general versus epidural anaesthesia in elderly patients. *Acta Anaesthesiol. Scand*; **27**:39.

Scott J. (1960). Post-operative disturbances in the aged. *Am. J. Surg*; **100**:38.

Sear J.W. *et al.* (1983). The effect of age on recovery. A comparison of kinetics of thiopentone and althesin. *Anaesth*; **38**:1158.

Sevitt G. (1973). The significance of fat embolism. *Brit. J. Hosp. Med*; **9**:784.

Seymour D.G., Pringle R. (1983). Post operative complications in the elderly surgical patient. *Gerontol*; **29**:262.

Simpson B.R. *et al.* (1961). The effects of anaesthesia and elective surgery on old people. *Lancet*; **ii**:889.

Strandgaard S. *et al.* (1973). Autoregulation of brain circulation in severe arterial hypertension. *Brit. Med. J*; **1**:507.

Welch K. (1959). Subdural haematoma following spinal anesthesia. *Arch. Surg*; **79**:49.

Wollner L. *et al.* (1979). Failure of cerebral autoregulation as a cause of brain dysfunction in the elderly. *Brit. Med. J*; **1**:1117.

# CHAPTER 7

# Medical aspects

## Patient examination

As much extra skill is required to examine an old person as for a small child. An unhurried history should be taken and the exact timing of acute as opposed to chronic complaints should be obtained because they are often mixed up in the history provided. A personal relationship and rapport may be developed while observing the patient's face, neck, arms, respiration, pulse and general well-being. There should then be a systematic examination of the back, chest, abdomen and legs of the patient, in that order. Inconsiderate or excessive bodily exposure should be avoided because it may cause much distress, especially to those who are shy. A full examination is essential as there is often no complaint of even the most obvious lesion, for example a breast lump or distended bladder. Finally, observing the patient's ability to sit, stand or walk may contribute to the diagnosis.

In later life there are certain conditions which are more common than at other times, for example dementia, osteoporosis and chronic lymphatic leukaemia. Conversely, infectious hepatitis, acute glomuerulonephritis, malignant hypertension and severe bronchitis are rare in the aged. There are also disorders to which the old are prone and for which there is diverse aetiology. These include autonomic system upsets, cerebral syndromes, falls, mental confusion, urinary or faecal incontinence, pressure sores and bone problems. A whole range or a combination of diseases is liable to afflict the old principally (Table 7.1).

One specific debilitating condition common in those over 70 years old is cranial (temporal or giant-cell) arteritis. It can present with headache, sudden poor sight, jaw claudication and pain with stiffness in the proximal limb muscles (polymyalgia rheumatica) and tender swollen scalp arteries with diminished

**Table 7.1**

*Diseases which principally afflict the elderly*

| Diseases with increased incidence in the elderly | Diseases mostly confined to the elderly |
| --- | --- |
| Tuberculosis | Osteoporosis |
| Septicaemia | Paget's disease |
| Pneumonia | Urinary and faecal incontinence |
| Coronary insufficiency | Dementia |
| Renal failure | Benign prostatic hypertrophy |
| Pulmonary embolism | Carcinoma of the prostate |
| Diabetes mellitus | Polymyalgia rheumatica |
| | Strokes |
| | Falls (common also in children) |
| | Parkinsonism |
| | Lymphatic leukaemia |

pulses, plus an ESR >50 mm/h. Urgent treatment with corticosteroids is necessary to prevent possible blindness. In doubtful circumstances, histology of a vessel biopsy is essential before or immediately after beginning steroid treatment.

There are other conditions which, although occurring throughout life, can present differently in the aged, for example diabetes, depression, fractures, myocardial infarction or heart failure, and those listed below.

1. 'Silent' abdominal surgical condition.
2. Infection without fever, tachycardia or leucocytosis.
3. Unexpected drug intoxication.
4. Malignant mass without local symptoms.
5. Pulmonary oedema without dyspnoea.
6. Pulmonary embolism without symptoms.
7. Myocardial infarction without pain.
8. Thyrotoxicosis with depression (apathy) and heart disease (auricular fibrillation). Only 50% of sufferers have thyroid swelling.
9. Depression without sadness.

## Nervous system

Where there is a short history of sudden onset of mental change, it may be a temporary state of confusion to which the old are prone. Where the changes take place slowly over many months, it may be progressive dementia. The distinction is made on the history and it is vital that this is accurate since the acute clouding of consciousness is often reversible while chronic dementia is seldom treatable but needs much attention as a management problem. Confusion can present as delirium, hallucinations, restlessness, violence or noisiness. Common precipitating causes are: *d*rug toxicity, *i*nfection (lung or urinary tract), *m*etabolic upset (diabetes or uraemia), *t*rauma, *o*xygen lack, and *p*sychological disturbance. These can be remembered by Gillis' mnemonic DIMTOP.

Strokes are a major cause of death and disability, and if 50 g of brain are lost by infarction, thrombosis or haemorrhage, it is likely that dementia will result. Only rarely can surgical evacuation of a blood clot help, but there may be improvement with the use of dexamethasone or mannitol if there is cerebral oedema. In the acute phase of a stroke, airway management and respiratory support with perhaps hyperventilation may be needed. For a patient living longer than 2 weeks after a stroke the prognosis for life is reasonably good and a considerable amount of rehabilitation is often possible. Dysphasia is a very disturbing condition for such patients and as their comprehension may be unaffected, one should always be discrete if they are belligerent while so desperate.

Some physicians recommend that elective operations should be postponed for at least 3 months after a cerebrovascular accident to avoid any recurrence. Although this advice is not as clearly statistically supported as is the risk of recurrence of coronary ischaemia, it is logical. It is important to know that transient ischaemic attacks, epilepsy, Stokes–Adams syndrome or postural hypotension can all lead to sudden incapacity perioperatively. Some authorities recommend for a transient ischaemic attack a thorough carotid artery investigation, with treatment if required and feasible, preoperatively. Orthostatic hypotension causing symptoms is not uncommon and in fact systolic blood pressure drops of 30 mmHg due to posture change occur in up to 9% of aged patients, and with certain drugs this condition is aggravated.

The incidence of depression and successful suicidal attempts increases steadily with ageing. Treatment with antidepressants is usually effective but unfortunately the condition is frequently missed because such patients often maintain a cheerful facade.

### Sight and sound

Concerning vision, the anaesthetist's knowledge of drug action in relationship to glaucoma is important, as is his or her understanding of nitrous oxide entrapment in cavities in relationship to the hearing loss in some old patients.

### Incontinence

Incontinence is a particular concern in the care of the elderly, when the frequency of the distressing symptom of urinary incontinence increases. The condition may be transient when it occurs as part of a general illness where there is clouding of consciousness, impairment of mobility, severe constipation or injudicious use of powerful loop diuretics. Established incontinence in the elderly can be due to the old person finding it increasingly difficult to inhibit the local reflexes which initiate bladder emptying. This results in the 'uninhibited bladder', associated with the urge to pass urine. Some patients develop an unstable bladder associated with urinary outflow obstruction which causes frequency, nocturia, urgency and urge incontinence. Stress incontinence occurs when the muscles of the pelvic floor are weakened, usually as a result of childbirth. Any cerebral or spinal lesion can, of course, present the predisposition of an uninhibited neuropathic bladder.

Faecal incontinence is similarly possible as a result of a neurogenic impairment of the gastrocolic reflexes, as in cerebrovascular disease or Alzheimer's disease, or due to any colonic pathology. But it is most commonly a symptom of constipation due to immobility. Some knowledge of these states is required by anaesthetists as they may find patients becoming incontinent after either anaesthesia (particularly conduction blocks) or pain therapy procedures.

### Pressure sores

There are two types of pressure sores: the shallow ones due to shearing forces can occur in fit patients; the deep ones are associated with unrelieved pressure and are most common in very ill patients (Fig. 7.1). It is important to understand that the normal capillary and venous pressures are 33 and 16 mmHg, respectively, and the pressures measured below the sacral and heel pressure points are usually 60–70 and 30–40 mmHg, respectively. Thus any immobility lasting more than 3 hours is dangerous, especially in the presence of hypotension. If there is a shearing or folding of the skin, necrosis will commence subcutaneously. It is thought that absolute risk factors are unconsciousness, dehydration and paralysis, the relative risk factors being age (older than 70), restricted mobility, incontinence, emaciation and redness over prominences. Observing those at risk closely allows early detection and preventative treatment of possible pressure sore areas. The Norton score relates to age, mental state, mobility, activity and continence,

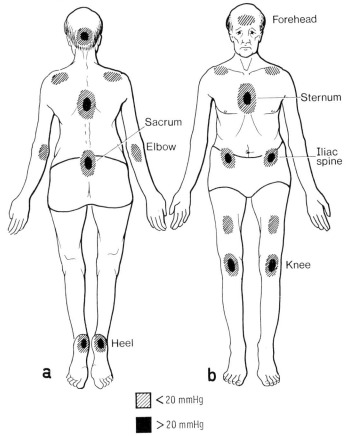

**Fig. 7.1** A diagram of the amount of pressure exerted in the supporting parts of the body in the supine (a) and prone (b) positions.

and if the score is less than 14, it indicates a need for special care—20% of hospital patients (see Appendix E3).

## Cardiovascular system

Because they will have run their course, valvular and pulmonary heart diseases are less common in older patients than cardiac ischaemia and hypertension. The last-mentioned can occur separately, or often together with atrial fibrillation or congestive cardiac failure. It is important to remember that the left jugular vein may be obstructed because the aorta and sternum can pinch the innominate vein. If the pressure in the right jugular vein is normal and the distension of the left subsides on deep respiration, the clinical impression of its relation to central venous pressure may be erroneous. One must avoid assigning importance to a neck bruit or apparent aneurysm when it is due to kinking of the right carotid artery with a short neck and dilated aorta. A left ventricular apex heave is observed normally in some fit old patients.

A systolic murmur is also a common physical finding, the significance of which may be difficult to understand. The anaesthetist needs to know whether a murmur is benign or indicates an important lesion. If a systolic murmur is very loud and accompanied by palpable thrill, with extension of the murmur towards the back, it is likely to be organic in origin. Innocent murmurs are, as a rule, of a blowing character, seemingly superficial and often varying with respiration. They are heard best in a small area to the left of the sternum near the second interspace. Diastolic murmurs are invariably pathological. In any case of doubt, a consultation with an expert is required. It is crucial to remember that up to two-thirds of older patients with myocardial infarction may not have chest pain. In fact the most common presenting symptoms are confusion, dyspnoea, hypotension, vomiting and weakness, later with the embolic sequelae.

Subacute bacterial endocarditis now seems to afflict more older than young patients, and the illness may present in a non-specific manner. A minimal heart lesion may be the origin of the condition, with a large range of subsequent bizarre features requiring repeated blood culture for confirmation of the diagnosis. Antibiotic cover for some operations, including minor dental and genitourinary, is always indicated for patients who have had endocarditis.

In youngish patients complete heart block is often due to infarction and has a poor prognosis. It must be remembered, however, that in the elderly heart block can be due to small fibrotic changes, and an artificial pacemaker is therefore often advisable as the prognosis may be good. Drugs which may cause heart block must be eliminated first, for example digoxin, quinidine, propranalol, or diuretics which cause hypokalaemia.

The management of mild, low or high arterial blood pressure is still a matter of debate. A small postural blood pressure drop is quite common in old patients, but symptomatically important postural hypotension (below 110 mmHg systolic) not only occurs on standing but is progressive with time. It must be recognised that apart from autonomic system failure, hypotension may well be due to drugs, bacteria or viral infection, myocardial infarction with low cardiac output or blood volume reduction through hyponatraemia or bleeding. If blood pressure is raised, then applying the Framingham study standard (>160/95 mmHg), more than two-thirds of ageing patients would be labelled hypertensive. It is usual to treat patients with diastolic pressure above 130 mmHg and associated with left ventricular hypertrophy or retinopathy. These patients are liable to congestive cardiac failure and cerebral haemorrhage and need urgent but not rapid treatment, usually first with a thiazide diuretic and propranolol and spironolactone or methyldopa. Patients with angina or dyspnoea on exertion should also have a trial of therapy.

Digitalis intoxication is quite common owing to its over-prescription, lack of recognition of small body mass, and poor excretion. The signs of intoxication include nausea, pulse rate less than 60/min, bigeminy, multifocal extrasystoli and arrhythmias. Indeed, the good effects of digitalis are not clear cut, whereas the bad effects are quite serious, and therefore it should be used sparingly in minimal effective doses.

## Blood

If anaemia is defined as a haemoglobin concentration of less than 13 g/dl in men and 12 g/dl in women, the frequency in general in the elderly in Britain is about 7%, but in geriatric wards it may be up to 40% of patients. The majority of anaemia may be accounted for by iron deficiency, megaloblastic changes, or chronic disease. Symptoms due to anaemia commonly develop when haemoglobin is <8 g/dl. Too often the old will accept symptoms of anaemia as inevitable and delay requesting medical attention. Congestive heart failure may be a presentation feature, as may mental symptoms. The standard treatments are, for iron deficiency anaemia, a daily oral dose of 150 mg of elemental iron, and for megaloblastic anaemia, hydroxycyanocobalamin 1000 µg weekly for a month and then 250 µg monthly for life. Where foliate deficiency is apparent, folic acid 5 mg t.d.s. is given. For anaemias due to chronic disease, treatment of the disease plus, in many instances, steroid therapy and folic acid are required.

It is important that blood tests should not be requested when a treatment decision is not liable to follow the reported findings. A full blood count may be combined with a second specimen of clotted blood from which the haematologist can (from the history and cell findings) investigate the serum $B_{12}$, foliate and ferritin levels, thus pinpointing any malabsorptive condition. The white count may indicate hidden chest or urinary infection or chronic leukaemia. Changes in plasma proteins in late life account for much higher ESR values in healthy people, thus patients with myocardial infarction or neoplastic disease may well have a 'normal' ESR. Low serum protein levels may be the first indication of poor nutrition, alcoholism, dementia or malabsorption, and may be the explanation of persistent pressure sores and ulcers or obscure leg oedema. Although a blood urea level is less useful than in earlier life owing to declining renal function, it may indicate correctable problems such as diarrhoea, vomiting, sweating or other dehydrating conditions.

The creatinine clearance rate is directly related to the elimination of some drugs and may be used with a nomogram to calculate dosage; it is also directly related to the incidence of renal failure after pyelography. At present, end-stage renal failure is not treated routinely with dialysis or transplantation in the elderly. In the light of survival, economics and rehabilitation, old patients should not be denied such treatment on the basis of age alone.

## Respiratory system

The vital capacity, the $FEV_{1.0}$ and the compliance are much reduced in the aged and in many instances basal crepitus will be heard on auscultation with no obvious aetiology (Fig. 7.2). Whenever there is impaired ventilation of the lungs, particularly in patients with a stroke or parkinsonism, this will be accentuated. The only consequence may be that the patient is apathetic and less mobile, with a raised pulse and respiratory rate. Lung infection may occur with little fever or rise in white blood count, but may cause confusion or heart failure. Empyema (now rare in young patients) may become apparent without fever or pleuritic pain, and drainage may be required for diagnostic purposes. When there is hypostatic (sometimes called 'terminal') pneumonia at the end of a chronic debilitating disease, treatment with antibiotics is of little avail. The decision about active treatment is therefore less important but must be on an individual basis as no general ruling can be valid. Severe emphysema is now more rare and mild in the very old,

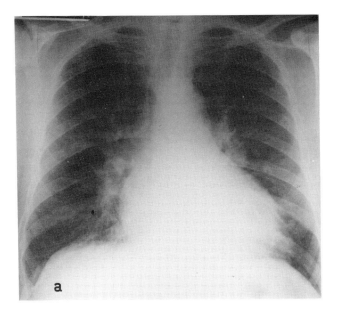

**Fig. 7.2(a)** A PA chest x-ray showing heart enlargement, perihilar opacification and evidence at the right base of interstitial oedema— 'Kerley B lines'.

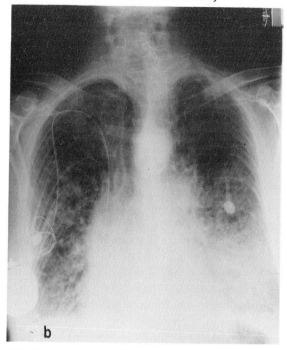

**Fig. 7.2(b)** Alveolar shadowing bilaterally extending from both hilar confluent at
the bases and compatible with acute pulmonary oedema. The pacemaker and
monitoring electrodes are also seen.

but the control of oxygen therapy is still essential because
smoking is still widespread and resultant hypercarbia not
uncommon.

Tuberculosis of the lung in the elderly is important and is
often the more rare miliary 'cryptic' disease, also there is a
need to avoid streptomycin owing to its propensity to produce
ear damage. In older patients lung carcinoma is less common in
men and less smoking related and its cure is so rare that
radiotherapy is usually recommended for symptoms only.


## Endocrine system

Much of the endocrine data changes yearly and is conflicting.
At present it is believed that pituitary growth hormone
excretion rate and the duration of secretion for each episode of
stress become less, but the pituitary–adrenal relationship is

unaltered with ageing. The renal clearance of iodine diminishes with age, but the extra circulating iodine is not cleared by the thyroid–that is, the rate of extraction of iodine decreases. Whereas plasma thyroxine ($T_4$) levels can remain constant, be increased or decreased, there is a constant or reduced triidothyronine ($T_3$) concentration with ageing: 1 in 25 geriatric patients has either thyrotoxicosis or myxoedema with few classical signs. Heart failure and atrial fibrillation are prominent, with a toxic thyroid and insidious mental and physical slowing with hypothyroidism, therefore the frequent use of screening tests is indicated. Parathyroid hormone levels fall slightly in men and rise in women, but the serum calcium level is slightly reduced in both sexes. Cortisol secretion rate declines, but serum levels are unchanged as the metabolic clearance rate is reduced. Aldosterone secretion rate declines, as does the circulating plasma level in response to fluid volume depletion. The response to adrenocorticotrophic hormone (ACTH) of the adrenal cortex and of the pituitary–adrenal axis to stimulation is questionably unaltered. It is important to realise that in the elderly endocrine dysfunction is atypical, therefore heightened awareness is needed for its recognition.

The term 'maturity onset' diabetes is used for a form in the elderly which is mild, develops slowly, and rarely causes ketosis. Often the plasma insulin level is normal or even raised and some authorities assign the carbohydrate disorder to a secondary role, indeed the most common first symptoms are cataracts, pruritis, claudication, gangrene, angina or peripheral neuropathy. The usual symptoms—polyuria, thirst, hunger, weight loss and coma—are more rare. As more than half of all diabetes commences in later life, mild conditions such as cramps and cold limbs, vision changes and bowel upsets require blood sugar level tests. A level of more than 100 + age mg/100 ml requires investigation and yearly follow-up. Any random blood sugar level greater than 11.1 mmol/l (200 mg/100 ml) or a fasting blood sugar greater than 7 mmol/l (126 mg/100 ml) confirms the presence of the metabolic disease. A glucose tolerance test produces levels of blood sugar 2 hours later greater than 6·6 mmol/l(120 mg/100 ml) in the majority of the elderly, and these borderline diabetics may be aggravated by any severe illness, even as far as becoming insulin dependent.

Individual treatment with diet, oral hypoglycaemics or insulin depends on the blood sugar levels and clinical and social factors. Rarer causes of raised blood sugar are important to the anaesthetist as they include thyrotoxicosis, phaeochromocytoma, brain damage, pancreatic disease and thiazide or steroid therapy.

The diagnosis of hypercalcaemia is not always obvious. Symptoms such as gastrointestinal upset, neurological problems and bone changes are often indefinite in the elderly; mild mental changes, lethargy or neurological evidence is particularly vague. A high level of suspicion requires biochemical screening to direct attention towards treatable hyperparathyroidism, other endocrine disorders or malignancy.

## When not to treat

The medical decision of when not to treat an old patient requires a fully history and examination, plus an assessment of the previous level of independence and health, motivation, mental state and life expectancy. The benefit of a treatment to the patient must be weighed against its hazards, which in the very old and frail may greatly depend on the standard of care. It is also important to modify the prognostic criteria used in the young for decisions in the elderly.

**Further reading**

Aderson K.E. *et al.* (1982). Prevention of pressure sores by identifying patients at risk. *Brit. Med. J*; **284**:1370.

Burley L.E. *et al.* (1979). Contribution from geriatric medicine within acute medical wards. *Brit. Med. J*; **11**:90.

Clark B.F., Campbell I.W. (1977). Direct addition of small doses of insulin to intravenous infusion in severe uncontrolled diabetes. *Brit. Med. J*; **2**:1395.

Cole W.H. (1970). Medical differences between the young and the aged. *J. Am. Geriatr. Soc*; **18**:589.

Denham M.J. (1972). The value of random blood glucose determination as a screening method for detecting diabetes mellitus in the elderly inpatient. *Age & Ageing*; **1**:55.

Gillis L.S. (1977). Confusion in the aged. *S. Afr. Med. J*; **51**:424.

Janbe D.H. *et al.* (1983). Successful treatment of middle aged and elderly patients with end stage renal disease. *Brit. Med. J*; **286**:2018.

Nichollis A.J. *et al.* (1984). Impact of continuous ambulatory peritoneal dialysis and treatment of renal failure in patients aged over 60. *Brit. Med. J*; **280**:18.

Steen P.A. *et al.* (1978). Cardiac reinfarction after anaesthesia and surgery. *J. Am. Med. Assoc*; **259**:2566.

Wright W.R. (1977). How to examine an old person. *Lancet*; **i**:1145.

CHAPTER 8

# Surgical aspects

## Collaboration of surgeon and geriatrician

Collaboration between surgeons and physicians who have a special interest in the elderly can be very beneficial. This was pioneered in Hastings in 1960 in orthopaedics and its use is increasing. Such cooperation can provide better preparation, postoperative care and, most of all, efficient effective rehabilitation. The special rehabilitation assistance geriatricians can provide is to the majority of patients whose future depends on management of their multiple pathology.

If the anaesthetist also has a concise understanding of the modern approach to geriatric surgery, he can contribute better to a team's efforts for the patient. In essence, with the elderly the surgeon aims to increase or preserve the patient's comfort more than to prolong life. The overall mortality of most operations is twice as great for the elderly compared with others, and doubles again if the procedure is not elective. Indeed, some urgent surgery has a mortality rate of 30% or more (see Appendix C). Regretfully, the mortality with minor operations is also greater for older subjects than for the young. Whereas the usual aim in surgery is to make the quality of life better for old patients, the result may be a cure, improvement or palliation of their condition. The aim has to be individualised, with a full assessment of the condition of each patient.

Clearly, to attempt always to cure is senseless, and staged procedures may be preferable in some circumstances. The skin of old patients is thin, with less collagen and fewer fibroblasts. This may relate to slower wound healing and more abdominal dehiscence (1% at 35 years and 5% at 75 years). Elasticity is less, so stretched skin does not recoil well and it may take 2 hours for skin pressed upon to regain its normal thickness. Time must be taken to give full attention to details in assessment and preoperative preparation, but with a minimum of unnecessary delay. One can fortify the patient's optimism for survival by preoperative education and by arranging a meeting with others who have had a similar lesion successfully operated upon. If perioperative care is immaculate (comparable to that extended to neonates), the old can stand the strain of operations of almost any magnitude.


**Nutrition**

Nutritional support in the malnourished may be valuable in providing stores of fuel and protein for the early postoperative period when endogenous resources are vital. Before a major operation, especially for cancer, a prognostic nutritional index can be arrived at as a guide to the depleted state. Reduced weight (>10% of normal body weight), albumin level (>3.5 mg/dl), or a lymphocyte count <1200/m$^3$ are indicators of the need for extra feeding. It is thought that only a small number of patients suffer sufficient protein-calorie malnutrition preoperatively to benefit from nutritional support, but studies to date are inconclusive. Anthropometric data such as arm circumference and triceps skinfold thickness correlate poorly with clinical pictures.

The carbohydrate store (as glycogen) is small and there is a need to provide essential fasting sugar levels for the brain, kidney and blood cells to function. Injury, including surgery and infection, will cause some metabolic increase but initially, with stress responses, proteinolysis dominates and nutritional manipulation is unhelpful. In fact, immediate postoperative feeding can burden the liver and kidneys, produce liver failure with fat overload, or cause heart strain. Recent work suggests that restricted nutritional support with an elemental content diet may suffice and be safer. A normal daily energy and nitrogen requirement is 126 kJ (30 kcal)/kg and 150 mg/kg respectively. The sodium (75 mmol) and potassium (50 mmol) requirements vary greatly with the disease present. An approximate daily basal requirement for other minerals by the intravenous route is phosphate 30 mmol, magnesium 15 mmol, calcium 7 mmol, zinc 150 μmol and iron 45 μmol. Trace element (copper, magnesium, fluoride and iodine) and vitamin (water and fat soluble) additions can be found in suitable commercial solutions. Beyond 5–7 days postoperatively the inevitable protein loss increases complications and mortality, so that artificial feeding becomes mandatory together with mobilisation and exercise to prevent unused muscles wasting.

## Abdominal surgery

Elective bowel cancer and biliary tract surgery are now often undertaken even when symptoms are not distressing, to avoid the high incidence of complications in those not operated upon. This has long been the case with peptic ulcers, hernias and vascular disease. Biliary tract operations are now a very common undertaking in the elderly. In the aged, acute infection of the gall bladder with or without operation has a high mortality (12%), and the majority of biliary tract disease is complicated. The average age for cholecystectomy in Britain is 62 years, and two-thirds of the elderly require bile duct exploration, compared with one-third of younger patients. Jaundice is most likely to be due to stone or tumour obstruction, whereas in younger patients it is more likely to be due to other causes. Twenty to thirty per cent of post-mortems carried out on those over 75 years old reveal gall-stones. Hepatitis (viral or serum) is rare in the elderly, as is acute pancreatitis.

Elective inguinal hernia repair should be freely advocated for old patients because emergency care increases mortality tenfold. Resection of the bowel for incarceration further doubles the mortality, but to replace unviable bowel ensures reoperation or subsequent death. Thus anaesthetists have to accept this difficult decision about bowel viability and the prolongation of anaesthesia it may require. When the bowel is resected the surgeon should empty it by milking contents to a large stomach or rectal tube or by threading a suction tube directly through a hole in the bowel. This helps relieve pressure on the lungs through the diaphragm, reduces the likelihood of a burst abdomen, and may ensure earlier peristalsis after the operation. A hernia may point to ascites from bowel cancer or an ovarian cyst, and urine retention or coughing may be contributing factors. It may be advisable to repair any hernia present when other straightforward operations are undertaken,

for example transurethral resection (TUR), retropubic prostatectomy or ovarian operations. Whether it is wise to repair
bilateral hernias together to avoid two operations depends on
whether the surgeon thinks recurrence is more common with a
double repair. Appendicitis is not common, but it is particularly dangerous in older patients as perforation is far more
frequent.

The excision of an oesophageal cancer is likely to produce an
immediate mortality of 10% and only 10% survival for 5 years.
For a fighting chance, anaemia, dehydration and malnutrition
must be corrected to some extent preoperatively and the
patient's physical condition before dysphagia must be discovered. Involvement of the bronchi, liver or brain should
preclude resection but Celestin intubation may provide the
palliation required. Two hazards of anaesthesia—pharyngeal
pouch and hiatus hernia—increase in incidence with ageing.
Stomach cancer is a desperate condition, often unresectable,
but requiring surgery for dysphagia and vomiting. Bleeding
from the gastrointestinal tract is ominous in the elderly—recent
medical and endoscopic advances in its treatment are
encouraging but surgical intervention may give the best chance
of survival. Peptic ulcers are not common, and conditions
which they may be mistaken for are critical to the anaesthetist,
for example myocardial infarction, aneurysm or mesenteric
infarction.

Bowel tumours are more common and less malignant (with a
better prognosis) in the old than in the young. Unfortunately,
however, diagnosis delay leads to more emergencies which
increases the operative mortality. Anaemia, hypoproteinaemia
and postoperative debility are frequent and can point to a
covert secondary spread of a tumour. Surgeons have limited
the use of colostomy for fear of management problems,
especially in the transverse colon, but primary resection is often
not possible in the aged. Concomitant poor vision, arthritis,
paraesthesia and poor domestic conditions all complicate the
management of a colostomy. However, with newer stomal
nursing care techniques and the advent of the stapling gun, the
surgical approach is changing rapidly. Certainly obstruction,
bleeding, mucus discharge, tenesmus and incontinence call for
possible operative relief, except where death is imminent.
Fulguration of rectal carcinomata may be useful in poor risk

patients. Diverticular disease is common in those over 50 years old and in the aged is as serious as cancer and requires radical excision when medical treatment fails. Prolapse of the rectum cannot be treated satisfactorily by the smaller procedure of Thiersch wiring, and anterior fixation is now advocated. Caecal or sigmoid colon volvulus is almost exclusively a disease of the elderly. Vague cramps and distension often require an abdominal x-ray to confirm this condition early enough for it to be treatable. There is a second peak in the incidence of Crohn's disease in the seventh decade.

## Urological surgery

The urology of the old primarily involves dealing with enlargement of the prostate, and cancer of the prostate or bladder. The transurethral resection of the prostate is preferable for 80% of patients, but retropubic operation may be retained for those with a very large prostates (>70 g) because it trebles the mortality (3% compared with 1%), as does acute urinary retention. The Helmstein pressure procedure (8 hours of bladder distention at diastolic blood pressure) is best for postradiation bleeding but worth a trial for a diffuse cancer of the bladder wall.

## Orthopaedic surgery

The incidence of fractures of the femur in patients over 60 years old doubles every 5 years for women and every 7 years for men. Osteomalacia, osteoporosis and tumour secondaries can all cause spontaneous fractures. With a femur fracture bed rest must be as limited as possible; only heart failure and poor diabetes control should briefly delay operation, or if death is imminent. Urgency is needed to circumvent all the ills of recumbency for the old, and the aim is to have the patient out of bed within 24 hours. At present pin and plate procedures are advisable for femur trochanteric fractures and a prosthesis for neck fractures to enable the earliest mobilisation. Other fractures to which the elderly are prone are those of the spine, distal radial and proximal humerus (areas in which there is cancellous bone).

There is an increasing amount of surgery for the treatment of painful and restricted joints. In order of frequency these joint replacements are required for the hip, knee, hand, elbow and shoulder. The need for arthrodesis and osteotomy is now quite infrequent. The factors which make a patient suitable for operation and the success rate for joint replacement are still undecided, but clearly surgical experience and immaculate asepsis are prime requirements. The overall mortality for total hip replacement averages 1–2%. The failure rate is 1–10% over 10 years. Sciatic or femoral nerves can be damaged by trauma or the insertion of the cement. Poor relaxation may cause further injuries or postoperative restlessness may be implicated in haematoma formation. During operations the refinements of venting the medullary cavity, use of a 'gun' when placing cement in bone or flooding of wounds with carbon dioxide may be helpful. Cement monomer liquid is highly inflammable and causes irritation to eyes and skin, so must be cautiously handled. An assessment of possible blood vessel disease before hip or knee joint replacement is sensible. Skin traction may lead directly, or through pressure areas, to bad ulceration.

## Vascular surgery

Abdominal aortic aneurysm presents at a mean age of 68 years. The operative mortalities for elective, acute and ruptured aortic aneurysms are approximately 5%, 20% and 40%, respectively. Acute aneurysms are said to present in 90% of patients with symptoms of pain and backache. The size is measurable with ultrasound (diameter >5.5 cm), and elective resection is indicated where there are the available staff and facilities. Resection, elective or emergency, has a good long-term effect, with the survival rate being only a little less than that expected for the same age group. With every laparotomy a full exploration is indicated to exclude the possibility of multiple pathology.

Arterial disease causes the greatest amount of disability for the elderly, particularly that of the brain, heart and legs. Surgical interventions in the form of carotid endarterectomy, coronary arterial bypass and grafting, clearing or replacing arteries are being employed for increasing numbers of old patients very successfully. Mesenteric thrombosis (arterial more than venous) increases with ageing and is catastrophic, so that heroic, and preferably early, operation is commended. When limb gangrene, or untreatable injury occurs, rapid amputation, with early provision of an artificial limb, is recommended to prevent pain and slow demise. While less than 40% of above-knee amputees will walk, nearly 80% of those with below-knee amputation will subsequently walk on an artificial limb. It has been found that older patients are less upset and cope better with amputation than do young patients.

## Antibiotics

Anaesthetists are being asked to administer systemic antibiotics at the induction of anaesthesia as the principles of their use are better established. The most successful prophylaxis is provided if a high blood level of the appropriate drug can be achieved at the time of contamination. The highest risk of infection is with colorectal surgery when neomycin, erythromycin, kanamycin, lincomycin or metronidazole are used separately or in combination. With biliary surgery, cephalosporins are effective and are essential in the aged with an obstructed or inflamed system. This is also the choice for gastric or womb surgery. Postoperative penicillin or metronidazole is used with amputations because of the risk of gas gangrene. With prosthetic joints or vessel grafts, flucloxacillin use is reasonable because subsequent infection is disastrous. Because dental work and cystoscopy cause bacteraemia, penicillin, erythromycin, gentamicin, amoxycillin or vancomycin is given for 48 hours to patients with defective hearts. An intravenous dose of antibiotics must not be given in less than 5 minutes in order to avoid the possible convulsive side-effects.

**Further reading**

*Metabolism*
Bastow M.D. *et al.* (1983). Benefits of supplementary tube feeding after fractured neck of femur: a randomised controlled trial. *Brit. Med. J*; **287**:1589.
Blichert-Toft M. *et al.* (1979). Influence of age on the endocrine-metabolic response to surgery. *Ann. Surg*; **190**(6):761.

Buzby G.P. *et al.* (1980). Prognostic nutritional index in gastrointestinal surgery. *Am. J. Surg*; **139**:160.

Chung B. *et al.* (1979). Nutritional deficiencies and nutritional support therapy in geriatric cancer patients. *J. Am. Geriatr. Soc*; **27**:491.

Collins J.P. *et al.* (1978). Intravenous amino acids and intravenous hyperalimentation as a protein sparing therapy after major surgery. A controlled clinical trial. *Lancet*; **i**:788.

Heatley R.V. *et al.* (1979). Preoperative intravenous feeding: a controlled trial. *Postgrad. Med. J*; **55**:541.

Holter A.R., Fischer J.E. (1977). The effects of perioperative hyperalimentation in patients with carcinoma and weight loss. *J. Surg. Res*; **23**:31.

Miller J.M. *et al.* (1982). Perioperative parenteral feeding in patients with G.I. carcinoma. *Lancet*; **i**:106.

Mullen J.L. *et al.* (1980). Reduction of morbidity and mortality by combined preoperative and postoperative nutritional support. *Ann. Surg*; **192**:604.

Oyama T. *et al.* (1980). Effect of anaesthesia and surgery on endocrine function in elderly patients. *Can. Anaesth. Soc. J*; **27**(6):556.

Sagar S. *et al.* (1979). Early postoperative feeding with elemental diet. *Brit. Med. J*; **1**:293.

*Vascular problems*

Bush H.L. Jr *et al.* (1977). Assessment of myocardial performance and optimal volume loading during elective abdominal aortic aneurysm resection. *Arch. Surg*; **112**(11):1301.

Bunker T.D., Taliff A.H.C. (1984). Uncontrollable bleeding under tourniquet. *Brit. Med. J*; **1**:1905.

Klenerman L., Lewis J.D. (1976). Incompressible vessels. *Lancet*; **i**:1811.

Lowe L.W. (1981). Venous thrombosis and embolism. *J. Bone & Jt Surg*; **63**:155.

Mann R.A., Bisset W.I. (1983). Anaesthesia and lower limb amputation. A comparison of spinal analgesia and general anaesthesia in the elderly. *Anaesth*; **38**(12):1185.

Modig J. *et al.* (1978). Systematic reactions to tourniquet ischaemia. *Acta Anaesthesiol. Scand*; **22**:609.

Pelletier L.C. *et al.* (1983). Open heart surgery in elderly patients. *Can. Med. Assoc. J*; **128**:409.

Pollard B.J. (1983). Fatal pulmonary embolism secondary to limb exsanguination. *Anesthesiol*; **58**:373.

Sigel B. *et al.* (1974). The epidemiology of lower extremity deep vein thrombosis in surgical patients. *Am. Surg*; **179**:278.

Storozzi C. *et al.* (1979). Disorders in peripheral arterial system in asymptomatic elderly. *Gerontol*; **25**:24.

# CHAPTER 9

# Common operation anaesthesia

## Introduction

There is little indication of how anaesthesia should be altered for old patients, apart from allowing for physiological and pharmacological changes by providing finesse in overall management. Some of the more common operations do, however, have specific problems which most anaesthetists recognise and treat in a standard way. The five most common operations in the elderly are cataract extraction, prostatectomy, hernia repair, cholecystectomy and hip pinning or replacement.

## Eye operations

Nearly half of all eye operations are carried out on patients over 65 years old, mostly for cataracts and detached retinas. These operations are not life-saving but are often associated with life-threatening concurrent conditions and are serious anaesthetic risks. Typically, heart failure, hypertension, angina or hypokalaemia may be present.

There seems little choice between a well-conducted local or general anaesthetic on the basis of mortality or morbidity, although local anaesthesia has been preferred for intraocular operations in patients with cardiovascular disease. The disturbing upset of routine and fears of eye surgery need to be ameliorated as far as possible by the preoperative interview and appropriate medication. Any chosen general anaesthetic method must provide stability of intraocular pressure, minimal bleeding and a 'still' eye. The sympathetic reflexes during intubation or the oculocardiac reflexes with eye manipulation are less obvious in the old. However, rotation of the eyeball for cataract extraction or iridectomy and pressure in the eye socket applied by a surgical pack or haematoma after enucleation are potent causes of reflexes. Monitoring is essential, and interruption of stimuli and intravenous atropine 0.3 mg are needed for severe bradycardia. Use of nitrous oxide with a narcotic and a non-depolarising muscle relaxant, artificial ventilation and a volatile agent to control hypertension, seems to give the most consistent success. If mannitol is used to control intraocular pressure, it must be done with caution in the elderly owing to the possibility of incipient heart failure.

Recent techniques make prolonged operations more common so that pressure points must be protected; also the good (unoperated) eye may have decreased tearing during anaesthesia so it must be assiduously protected with both local and general anaesthesia. The cornea must be protected carefully because with ageing it becomes less sensitive and more liable to injury.

Long-acting anticholinesterase drugs (ecothiopate or demecarium) are used locally in the eye and may interact with relaxants. Suxamethonium raises intraocular pressure for about 6 minutes so should not be used with closed angle glaucoma, a perforating eye injury, or immediately before an orbit is to be opened. The control of excess intraocular pressure involves hyperventilation, hypotension, head-up position and perhaps retrobulbar block, mannitol, lignocaine or propranolol intravenously. If halothane is used, a maximum of 10 ml 1/100 000 adrenaline (0.1 mg) is permissible for local haemostasis. To reduce the occurrence of postoperative confusion, one eye should be uncovered, ambulation encouraged and a normal diet quickly restored (ketamine should not be used). Intramuscular cyclizine 25 mg 6-hourly, or perphenazine 2.5 mg 12-hourly are the preferred antiemetics. There is a need to be aware of the recently discovered association of autonomic dysfunction, glaucoma and diabetes.

## Prostatectomy

Whilst it is usually expected that there may be major blood loss with a suprapubic prostatectomy, it should also be recognised that blood loss with transurethral prostatic resections is also significant. The measurement or assessment of the amount of blood lost is difficult because of bladder irrigation.

Also, the usual prostatectomy patient's ability to withstand a major blood loss is often limited. Nevertheless, any mortality from blood loss should be as critically reviewed as it would be with tonsillectomy today. Early recognition and correction of hypovolaemia must be a priority of staff involved in the care of these patients. Apart from the problem of haemorrhage in the old man requiring this operation, it has long been recognised that fluid may be absorbed rapidly from the distended bladder through injured veins and this can cause serious fluid overloading and electrolyte changes (in 2–4% of patients). The amount of fluid absorbed depends on the number of venous sinuses opened, the duration of the exposure, and the pressure within the bladder being greater than the venous pressure. A volume of 20 ml/min or more may be absorbed. A solution of glycine is commonly used, up to 2.1%; it is isotonic, non-haemolytic and does not disperse high-frequency current as it is non-electrolytic and has good optical properties. It can, however, cause ammonia intoxication if sufficient is absorbed intravenously. When an isotonic glucose solution is used for irrigation there is a greater drop in serum sodium and a considerable rise in blood glucose, and these changes will become apparent as confusion, headache, nausea, retching, bradycardia, raised blood pressure and dyspnoea, cyanosis or even finally blood pressure drop and cardiac arrest. Under general anaesthesia the signs are masked and the condition may only be evident from pulse rate and blood pressure changes or postoperatively by delayed recovery.

Preventive measures are to ensure that the operating time is limited, that the tissue excision extends to the capsule of the prostate rather than dividing many sinuses, and that the pressure within the bladder is not above 70 cm $H_2O$. Of course, it is essential not to give more hypotonic solution intravenously. As it is common to force diuresis with this procedure, hyponatraemia is usual but short lived. A persistent blood sodium level of less than 125 mmol/l will produce clinical signs. If there are cerebral or cardiovascular signs, it is important to monitor the central venous pressure, to give hypertonic saline (1.8%), a diuretic (20% mannitol/250 ml) and calcium as an inotropic agent. For the severely affected peritoneal dialysis may be required. For prostatectomy meticulously conducted general anaesthesia can lead to haemorrhage as limited as that provided by hypotensive or conduction block techniques. About 1% of patients may get a perforated bladder, and some anaesthetists therefore favour regional anaesthesia because the patient's complaint of pain may lead to earlier recognition of this complication. Another complication with a similar incidence is fibrinolysis activated by substances released from the prostate, and this may be countered by episilon aminocaproic acid. This drug is given prophylactically by a few anaesthetists.

A possibility of bacteraemia and the electrical hazards, especially in a patient with a pacemaker, complete the list of problems.

## Hernia repair

Most hernias should be repaired because of the great discomfort they cause, as much as for the future hazards they present. Local analgesia can provide ideal operating conditions with minimal risk. However, the obese, fearful or irrational patient may be unsuitable for local analgesia, and the possible need for a major procedure (with possible wide peritoneal opening) rather than a limited one is another contraindication.

Aided early mobilisation, individualised analgesia and extra respiratory care are essential postoperatively to ensure limited morbidity. Proper preparation and organised home care should enable admission to be reduced to 24 hours for many patients.

## Cholecystectomy

Conduction anaesthesia can be preferred for all the operations mentioned in this chapter, but it is least satisfactory for this major upper abdominal procedure. Because it is so common and often now entails only short (5 days) in-patient care, the dangers of this operation must not be underestimated. A large deep wound inflicted in the middle of a patient for the delicate dissection of vital structures in a position where reflexes are easily initiated cannot be treated lightly.

A general anaesthetic combination of minimal 'sleep dose' intravenous induction with light level inhalation maintenance supplemented by intravenous analgesic and muscle relaxant is the most common and widely used method at present. For anaesthetists with limited experience, this method can be advocated for almost every undertaking in elderly patients, and a critique of it merely directs us to its perfection.

Awareness is possible, but rare in the elderly, and good control of the agents is therefore required to ensure changed perception at all times. Perfected premedication, continuous monitoring and ensured unconsciousness at the beginning and end of the procedure are essential. With the artificial controlled ventilation required, the need to minimise the cardiovascular and respiratory physiological trespass is evident—the more so the more diseased the patient. Isovolaemia, eucapnia and limited intrathoracic pressure are aimed at by means of clinical acumen and measurement. Well-applied routine endotracheal intubation is beneficial and its ill-effects can be limited. A refined technique and care of endotracheal intubation are needed, for example humidification of nasal bypassed gases and cuff pressure control.

Adequate postoperative ventilation is most prone to be neglected in the vulnerable elderly. The causes are variable, but proper application of a peripheral nerve stimulator, use of drug antidotes, and continued endotracheal intubation and controlled ventilation for any indications ensure effective care.

## Hip pinning and prosthesis

As these are now common and increasingly frequent operations, their associated high mortality and morbidity are a cause for concern. A number of papers have indicated that mortality may be halved by the use of conduction anaesthesia (6% in pooled data), and there is evidence that general anaesthesia may adversely affect fibrinolysis and blood coagulation. There is also a suggestion that controlled ventilation and relaxant may adversely influence thrombosis and mortality.

Mortality is most frequent on the 6th and 18th postoperative days and strongly relates to the incidence of deep vein thrombosis. Deep vein thrombosis is reported in 45–70% of these operations, depending on whether the inaccurate clinical diagnosis or the reliable fibrinogen uptake test is used. Almost inevitably, the femoral vein is occluded by adduction and external rotation of the leg during prosthetic hip replacement. Regional anaesthesia is said to reduce the blood loss by half during these operations as well as to reduce the frequency of postoperative deep vein thrombosis (from 55% to 28% in one study). Unfortunately it is not yet clear which is the most effective prophylactic method owing to the many varying regimens applied by different surgeons. Anticoagulation prophylaxis seems justified, despite the extra risk of bleeding, because it does appear to reduce the incidence of pulmonary embolism.

During the operation, extensive preparation of the femur may cause bradycardia, extrasystole or cardiac arrest, and a consistent fall in arterial oxygen tension. This has been blamed on the acrylic cement, the high pressures within the medullary cavity when inserting the cement or the prosthesis, or the inherent poor condition of most patients. The polymerisation of the monomer is associated with high temperature and this, or any intravascular monomer, can cause hypotension, tachycardia and a large increase in cardiac output. It is suggested that the cement should only be used after it has reached a stiff consistency to reduce the amount of monomer entering the circulation. The pressures created in the bone will force bone cavity contents (air, marrow fat, thromboplastic products) into thin-walled or already damaged vessels, leading to a pulmonary embolic syndrome.

After any major hip operation, knee replacement or leg fracture, an incidence of fat embolism is evident. The indefinite signs and symptoms occur 24–48 hours after operation or injury. Restlessness and delirium with headache and irritability may be followed by stupor, coma and shock. Fever, tachypnoea, petechiae on the shoulders or white retinal exudates may be produced. Oxygen, digoxin, aminophylline, heparin and intravenous alcohol are the agents suggested to combat the complex lung damage. In some centres, the $Pao_2$ is monitored daily and if petechiae or reduced oxygen levels occur, steroids are given as a routine treatment (methylprednisolone 1 g t.d.s.). In some instances intensive care with ventilatory support may be required.

The main requirements in all this work are careful fluid therapy and transfusion, an increase of inspired oxygen before cement or prosthesis insertion (or tourniquet release), and prolongation of oxygen administration and monitoring for 48 hours postoperatively.

**Further reading**

*Eye*

Adams A.P., Fordham R.M. (1973). General anesthesia in adults. *Int. Ophthalmol. Clin*; **13**:83.

Donion J.V. Jr (1980). Local anaesthesia for ophthalmic surgery: patient preparation and management. *Ann. Ophthalmol*; **12**(10):1183.

Karhunen U., Jonn G. (1982). A comparison of sensory function following local and general anaesthesia for the extraction of senile cataract. *Acta Anaesthesiol. Scand*; **26**:291.

Karhunen U., Orko R. (1981). Nausea and vomiting after local anaesthesia for cataract extraction in elderly female patients — effect of droperidol premedication. *Ophthalmic Surg*; **12**(11):810.

Mapstone R., Clark C. V. (1985). Prevalence of diabetes in glaucoma. *Brit. Med. J*; **291**: 93.

Martin J.J. *et al.* (1976). The efficacy of general anaesthesia for cataract surgery. *Ophthalmic Surg*; **7**(3):89.

*Prostate*

Abrams P.H. *et al.* (1982). Blood loss during transurethral resection of prostate. *Anaesth*; **37**:71.

Erlik *et al.* (1968). Prostatic surgery and the cardiovascular patient. *Brit. J. Urol*; **40**:53.

Lerner S. (1973). Suppression of demand pacemaker by transurethral electrosurgery. *Anesth. Analg*; **52**:703.

McGowan S.W., Smith G.F.N. (1980). Anaesthesia for transurethral prostatectomy and comparison of spinal intradural analgesia with two methods of general anaesthesia. *Anaesth*; **35**:847.

Osborn D.E. *et al.* (1980). Fluid adsorption during transurethral resection. *Brit. Med. J*; **281**:1549.

Roesch R.R. *et al.* (1983). Ammonia toxicity resulting from glycine absorption during transurethral resection of the prostate. *Anesthesiol*; **58**:579.

*Hernia*

Guillen J., Aldrete J.A. (1970). Anaesthetic factors influencing morbidity and mortality of elderly patients undergoing inguinal herniorrhaphy. *Am. J. Surg*; **42**:859.

Ponka J.L., Brush B.E. (1974). Experience with the repair of groin hernia in 200 patients aged 70 or older. *J. Am. Geriatr. Soc*; **22**:18.

Tingwald G.R., Cooperman M. (1982). Inguinal and femoral hernia repair in geriatric patients. *Surg. Gynecol. Obstet*; **154**(5):704.

*Hip*

Aldrete J.A. *et al.* (1967). Anaesthesia factors in surgical management of hip fractures. *J. Trauma*; **7**:811.

Alexander J.P., Barron D.W. (1978). Clinical considerations in anaesthesia for hip arthroplasty. *Anaesth*; **33**:748.

Alexander J.P., Barron D.W. (1979). Biochemical disturbances associated with total hip replacement. *J. Bone & Jt Surg*; **61B**:101.

Alho A. *et al.* (1978). Corticosteroids in patients with a high risk of fat embolism syndrome. *Surg. Obstet. Gynaecol*; **147**:358.

Amaranath L. *et al.* (1975). Relation of anesthesia to total hip replacement and control of operative blood loss. *Anesth. Analg*; **54**:641.

Berry F.R. (1977). Analgesia in patients with fractured shaft of femur. *Anaesth*; **32**:576.

Cooke E.D. *et al.* (1977). Intravenous lignocaine in prevention of deep vein thrombosis after elective hip surgery. *Lancet*; **ii**:797.

Dandy D.J. (1971). Fat embolism following prosthetic replacement of femoral head. *Injury*; **3**:85.

Davis F.M. *et al.* (1980). Deep vein thrombosis and anaesthetic technique in emergency hip surgery. *Brit. Med. J*; **2**:1528.

Davis F.M., Laurenson V.C. (1981). Spinal anaesthesia or general anaesthesia for emergency hip surgery in elderly patients. *Anaesth. Int. Care*; **9**(4):352.

Devas M.B. (1974). Geriatric orthopaedics *Brit. Med. J*; **1**:190.

Ellis R.H., Mulvein J. (1973). Cardiovascular effects of methylmethacrylate. *Anesthesiol*; **38**:102.

Ellison N., Mull T.D. (1974). Unique anesthetic problems in the elderly patient coming to surgery for fracture of the hip. *Ortho. Clin. N. Am*; **5**(3):493.

Hole A. *et al.* (1980). Epidural versus general anaesthesia for total hip arthroplasty in elderly patients. *Acta Anaesthesiol. Scand*; **24**:279.

Keith I. (1977). Anaesthesia and blood loss in total hip replacement. *Anaesth*; **32**:444.

Koide M. *et al.* (1974). Anesthetic experience with total hip replacement. *Clin. Ortho. Related Res*; **99**:78.

McLaren A.D. *et al.* (1978). Anaesthetic techniques for surgical correction of fractured neck of femur. A comparative study of spinal and general anaesthesia in the elderly. *Anaesth*; **33**(1):10.

Martin V.C. (1977). Hypoxaemia in elderly patients suffering from fractured neck of femur. *Anaesth*; **32**(9):852.

Modig J. *et al.* (1975). Arterial hypotension hypoxaemia during total hip replacement. *Acta Anaesthesiol. Scand*; **19**:28.

Modig J. *et al.* (1983). Role of extradural and of general anaesthesia on fibrinolysis and coagulation after total limb replacement. *Brit. J. Anaesth*; **55**:625.

Nightingale P.J., Marstrand T. (1981). Subarachnoid anaesthesia with bupivacaine for orthopaedic procedures in the elderly. *Brit. J. Anaesth*; **53**:369.

Sanui K. (1979). Intraoperative haemodynamic changes during total knee replacement. *Anesthesiol*; **50**:239.

Sculco T.P., Ranawat C. (1975). The use of spinal anaesthesia for total hip replacement arthoplasty. *J. Bone & Jt Surg*; **57A**:173.

Spreadbury T.H. (1980). Anaesthetic technique for surgical correction of fractured neck of femur. A comparative study of ketamine and relaxant anaesthesia in elderly women. *Anaesth*; **35**:208.

Stamatakis J.D. *et al.* (1978). Femoral vein thrombosis and total hip replacement. *Brit. Med. J*; **1**:1031.

Thompson C.E. *et al.* (1978). Hypotensive anesthesia for total hip replacement. *Anesthesiol*; **48**:91.

White I.W.C., Campbell W.A. (1980). Anaesthesia for surgical correction of fractured femoral neck. A comparison of three techniques. *Anaesth*; **35**:1107.

Wickstom I. *et al.* (1982). Survival of female geriatric patients after hip fracture surgery. A comparison of 5 anaesthetic methods. *Acta Anaesthesiol. Scand*; **26**(6):607.

Wilcock G.K. (1981). A comparison of total hip replacement in patients aged 64 years or less or 70 years or over. *Gerontol*; **27**:85.

# CHAPTER 10

# Diagnostic and therapeutic procedures

## Introduction

The anaesthetist is not asked to assist in many diagnostic procedures involving the elderly. With modern investigative techniques and apparatus and the inherent stoicism of older patients, it is rare for analgesia to be required beyond that which is given by the physician or surgeon.

## Endoscopy

Fibreoptic endoscopy of the urinary bladder, bowel or bronchi usually requires only sedation for the majority of patients, and in many cases intravenous diazepam is used. The anaesthetist should advise on the dose, particularly for sick patients. Adequate time should be allowed for the full effect to be observed, and the increased incidence of thrombosis of the injected vein with diazepam with ageing should be borne in mind. To avoid this latter sequelae, diazepam in an emulsive form (Diazemul) is preferable. Alternatively, dilution and administration through a major vein with an infusion may be helpful. Any adjuvant topical anaesthetic should be applied in a non-toxic dose and sufficient time allowed for its full action. After the administration of such a long-acting drug as diazepam, it is necessary to have proper postoperative observation. When general anaesthesia is required for endoscopy it is crucial that the full risk of the anaesthetic be recognised.

An experienced anaesthetist should be responsible for postponement or cancellation of the procedure as required when there is serious risk or an incident during the undertaking. The importance of a diagnostic procedure lies in its relation to future therapy. The occurrence of damage during instrumentation must always be recognised as a possibility. The less obvious signs of complications in the elderly and the dire consequence of delayed treatment must be understood.

## Vascular work

The placement of an epicardial and occasionally an intravenous pacemaker will require general anaesthesia. The vulnerability of patients requiring this operation and the irritation of the myocardium that can occur make this a risky procedure necessitating awareness of all the pacemaker patient's problems. Proper monitoring and recovery observation are mandatory. Occasionally block of peripheral nerves may facilitate vascular diagnostic decisions. (These are described in Chapter 11.) Angiography of major vessels supplying the brain and limbs is now commonly undertaken because corrective surgery may be available. Local anaesthesia or general anaesthesia is needed for the major neck or arm vessel studies, but in the more common lower limb investigations a lumbar epidural anaesthetic may be preferable.

## Epidural block

Single-dose lumbar epidural block to the level of L1 (produced by 0.5% bupivacaine up to 20 ml) is satisfactory for descending aorta and leg vessel angiography. It may be more suitable than general anaesthesia in the difficult circumstances which may obtain in a radiology department. For the Helmstein's procedure (distension of the urinary bladder for 7–8 hours), it is usual to use continuous epidural block to the T10 level. To obtain successful painlessness for this duration requires early top-up of the epidural block and expert nursing care with psychological support and, occasionally, extra sedation. This is most likely to be perfected in a recovery or intensive care unit where the nursing staff is more concentrated.

For many back pain problems, with or without sciatic pain, a lumbar or caudal epidural injection of fluid, local anaesthetic or steroids appears beneficial for some patients. The success rate may be enhanced by concurrent physiotherapy. A mixture of lignocaine 1.5%, 10 ml, saline 0.9%, 10 ml, and Depo-Medrone 80 mg, and hydrocortisone 50 mg has stood the test of wide use with minimal side-effects. Such epidural injections may be said to be principally to relieve pain, but local epidural analgesia is included in this chapter because it can also be used diagnostically. Block of the sympathetic system indirectly in this way may be used for vasospastic states when the vasodilatation response can be assessed by blood flow, temperature or galvanic response. Local, temporary or semipermanent block of S2 unilaterally by the trans-sacral route may be beneficial with bladder neck spasm or carcinoma pain.

## Lumbar sympathetic block

In the elderly a common therapeutic block employed is lumbar sympathetic chemical blockade. Because of the old patient's poor general condition, this may be the only available therapy for rest pain, trophic ulcers, oedema or impending gangrene of the legs. With the possible exception of aspirin, no drug has been proven to improve peripheral blood flow, so many expensive prescribed remedies are wasted. The results of this block are often clinically favourable but there is no accepted objective assessment of the different techniques.

First, the patient is seen for assessment of suitability, preparation, and a full explanation about the undertaking. Any blood dyscrasia, anticoagulation therapy or local sepsis is a mandatory contraindication to this block. The consent signature should be obtained from the patient after a second explanation of the procedure and its expected results. Time for extended consideration and to formulate questions is essential with aged patients. Premedication is rarely indicated but fasting should be ordered for 4 hours preoperatively. Any sedation is safer and more controlled if given by the intravenous route during the procedure. The blood pressure should be monitored perioperatively.

Good positioning of the patient is crucial and the affected side to be injected should be uppermost, with the spine straightened as much as possible by radiotranslucent pillows. Some flexion of the knees and mechanical brackets will help support the patient. Flexion of the arms is required for x-ray

purposes. Image intensification x-ray and radio-opaque injections are essential for the correct placement of the block
solution. Whereas in young patients it is advisable to have a
preliminary injection of a local anaesthetic, in the elderly it
may be less traumatic and desirable to undertake the procedure
with long-acting chemicals (such as phenol) where there is no
previous indication of the block's likely success.

Both lateral and posterior–anterior projection views with the
image intensifier are required, and an experienced radio-
grapher is helpful in obtaining good views (Fig. 10.1). Full
aseptic precautions are used and the landmarks are carefully
drawn with a sterile pen. The distance from the spines of the

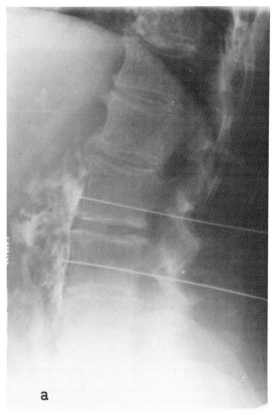

a

**Fig. 10.1(a)** A lateral x-ray image of needle placement and injected opaque media,
anterior to the bodies of the 2nd and 3rd lumbar vertebrae.

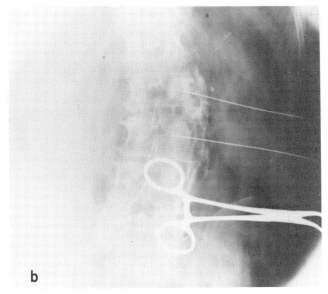

**Fig. 10.1(b)** A posterior/anterior image of the x-ray of needle placement and injected opaque media anterolateral to the body of the 2nd and 3rd lumbar vertebrae. A slight scoliosis is produced by an inflatable cushion below the patient.

vertebrae to the skin entry point is usually 8–10 cm; 22-gauge 15-cm long needles are most commonly used for this block, and rubber depth markers on the needles are helpful. The choice of levels to be blocked (L2, L3 or L4) depends on the position of the lesion on the limb, or on the practicality of the injection. Injection of air on the needle point reaching the anterior vertebral body may assist radiographic identification of the correct position. However, the main indication is the distribution of the radio-opaque dye in both projections (x-rays). Three millilitres of 0.5% bupivacaine are injected first. Observation of the ability to move the toes after 3 minutes will indicate any subarachnoid spread. This preliminary local anaesthetic injection will also make the phenol injection painless. For prolonged block, 3 ml of 7.5% phenol at each vertebral level is the method of choice. For 15–20 minutes after injection the patient is kept in the same lateral position to reduce seepage of the agent laterally. Blood pressure is measured every 20 minutes for 2 hours postinjection and for 2 hours after the patient gets out of bed. In the presence of some dysautonomia, the block may produce a significant postural hypotension. Only one side is done at a time but the opposite side may be injected 2–3 weeks later.

Rare complications of the block are somatic nerve block or irritation, subarachnoid tap, blood vessel or kidney puncture. The commonest of these is an L2 neuralgia which is self-limiting and can be controlled by applying a transcutaneous electrical nerve stimulator.

For upper abdominal carcinoma pain, coeliac plexus block may be carried out in the same manner. However, up to 100 ml of 50% alcohol may be needed to block all the nerve's ramifications, and a bilateral injection may best be given in the prone position. With the injection level at L1, a pneumothorax is an added hazard. A block of splanchnic nerves bilaterally at the T12 level may be successful when the coeliac plexus is displaced by tumour.

## Electroconvulsive therapy (ECT)

Many anaesthetists are involved in providing unconscious-ness and relaxation for the administration of electroconvulsive therapy. The main indication for this treatment is endogenous depression, which is common in the elderly. In Northwick Park Hospital (England) the incidence of ECT in various age groups is approximately as follows.

$$<65 \text{ years} = 60\%$$
$$66–75 \text{ years} = 20\%$$
$$>75 \text{ years} = 20\%$$

The frailty of many of these patients, with junior staff undertaking their care in a unit situated away from other anaesthetic help, may create a high-risk situation. It is therefore important that there is proper assessment and monitoring of such patients and full resuscitation facilities.

Myocardial infarction or a cerebrovascular accident, raised intracranial or intraocular pressure, and thrombophlebitis are contraindications to ECT. The routine use of atopine pre-treatment is not helpful. Proper recovery facilities and nursing

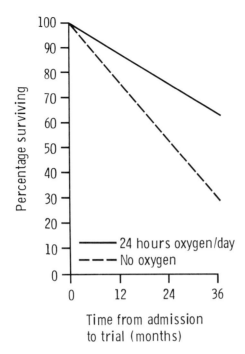

**Fig. 10.2** The percentage of patients surviving in relationship to time, with and without the administration of oxygen, when suffering from chronic obstructive airways disease.

care are as important in this work as they are following surgical anaesthesia.


## Oxygen therapy

Oxygen therapy in the homes of patients with chronic bronchitis and emphysema is being more widely advocated. Patients with cor pulmonale who have a $Pao_2$ <50 mmHg (6.6 kPa) may have their polycythaemia reduced and the progression of pulmonary hypertension prevented by oxygen therapy. It would be unreasonable to provide long-term oxygen supplies to those who smoke and thus have a carboxyhaemoglobin >3% (and who risk burning themselves while receiving oxygen). Such treatment may extend the life of some patients (Fig. 10.2), and it also considerably reduces their distress.

The provision of a machine to dissociate the oxygen from the air (an oxygen concentrator) is more sensible and economic in the long term than providing gas in cylinders. The cost of providing oxygen in the long term by concentrator is approximately one-fifth of that for cylinder delivery. Patients need a 1–3 l/min oxygen supply to nasal prongs (enriching air breathed), and therefore humidification is not essential. If the $Pao_2$ is raised to approximately 70 mmHg (9.3 kPa) and controlled at that level, the theoretical risk of dangerous carbon dioxide retention does not occur in practice. There is evidence of hypoxia and mild hypocapnia in the acute and recuperative stages of hemiplegia, and therefore oxygen therapy may be beneficial, in hospital or at home, in preserving brain tissue in a patient suffering from a stroke.

## Temperature management

Anaesthetists may be also asked for advice concerning the management of a patient with hypothermia or hyperthermia —conditions which occur relatively commonly in the elderly.

Hypothermia treatment should be undertaken in an intensive care unit if the patient's temperature is below 35°C. Gradual warming is advised by means of warmed blankets, with the aim of raising the temperature by 0.5°C per hour. Immersion of one limb only in warm water (40–44°C) and prevention of heat loss with a blanket in a warm environment give controlled rewarming. The rectal temperature is used to monitor the rate of temperature rise. A metalised plastic space blanket can be used to speed the temperature rise should it be too slow. A rapid increase of temperature must be avoided because serious hypotension may ensue. Below 32°C ventricular fibrillation which is resistant to defibrillation is a considerable risk, and therefore the ECG should be monitored at all times. If there is cardiac arrest, a prolonged attempt at resuscitation is indicated because the low temperature may protect the vital organs and favour full recovery. Oxygen administered with a heated humidifier through a closed circuit may assist temperature rise. Analysis of blood gases should be routine, applying the corrections for their measurement at 37°C. Because bronchopneumonia is a common occurrence, x-ray of the chest and antibiotic coverage should be routine. Warm gastric or colonic lavage, warm intravenous infusion, warm mediastinal irrigation, partial cardiac bypass and peritoneal dialysis can all be undertaken with fluids at 38–43°C. Pulmonary oedema and hypotension during the warming are common, and a 50% mortality is often reported. Therefore a highly organised aggressive management in intensive care conditions may be worth a trial study. Moderate (28–32°C) or severe (<28°C) hypothermia, especially if circulatory or respiratory failure, cardiac dysrhythmias or diabetic coma occurs, requires intensive care for core rewarming.

*Intensive care of hypothermia*

1. Protect airway and ventilate.
2. Administer controlled oxygen therapy.
3. Monitor ECG, arterial blood pressure, central venous pressure and core temperature.
4. Give warm intravenous fluids and inhaled gas.
5. Measure serum potassium, blood sugar, blood gases and pH at frequent intervals.
6. Undertake peritoneal dialysis.
7. Give extracorporeal heat exchange.
8. Give intravenous hydrocortisone 100 mg 6-hourly.
9. Give intravenous broad-spectrum antibiotics.
10. Give tri-iodothyroxine 10 µg 8-hourly for comatose myxoedematous patients.

Previous aggressive care has entailed rapid rewarming in general ward conditions and has proved disastrous.

Hyperthermia has an even greater mortality rate than hypothermia. The treatment is gradual cooling with intensive care monitoring, paying particular attention to fluid, electrolyte and acid-base balance. The recommended treatment is immersion in a cold bath or tepid water/alcohol sponging—2 litres of 0.5 normal saline plus dextrose intravenously in 1 hour followed by 1 litre 4-hourly, with potassium addition when the urine output improves, and then chlorpromazine in small increments to cause peripheral vasodilation and provide sedation.

**Aggressive patients**

Chlorpromazine intramuscularly may be used to control violent, aggressive patients, for example those who are demented or confused. When reassurance is of no avail, haloperidol or droperidol 10 mg intramuscularly or, for maintaining control, a 0.8% solution of chlormethiazole, may be required.


**Herpes zoster and amputations**

Although it has not been verified by study, some anaesthetists claim they can contribute therapeutically or prophylactically to patients with herpes zoster and amputation problems. Thus, if patients with herpes zoster are treated by sympathetic block during the acute phase, it is possible that postherpetic neuralgia (which is so common and distressing in old patients) would occur less often.

The block chosen should be the most practical. Therefore for head and neck lesions this will be the cervical stellate ganglion, for the thoracic region the paravertebral somatic of the appropriate level, and for lower abdominal and lower limb the lumbar epidural block. These blocks should be maintained for 3 or 4 days or repeated on two or three occasions during the acute phase. They can lead to rapid clearing of the weeping excoriating lesions and relief of acute pain.

In the case of amputation, it is suggested that a continuous somatic block of the painful area due to be amputated will lead to a reduced incidence of postamputation phantom limb pain. This may be achieved by continuous brachial block, lumbar, caudal or spinal injections. Also, if nerves are frozen at the time of amputation, their involvement in phantom activity may be aborted, but this is also unproven. It is possible that paravertebral somatic or intercostal nerve block for relief of the pain of fractured ribs may also have a therapeutic role because the underlying lung dysfunction may then be less severe and less prolonged.

**Further reading**

Cousins M.J. *et al.* (1979). Neurolytic lumbar sympathetic blockade; duration of denervation and relief of rest pain. *Anaesth. Int. Care*; **7:**121.

Haas A. *et al.* (1967). Respiratory function in hemiplegic patients. *Arch. Phys. Med. Rehab*; **48:**174.

James C.D.T., Little T.F. (1976). Regional hip blockade. *Anaesth*; **31:**1060.

Marks R.J. (1984). Electroconvulsive therapy: physiological and anaesthetic considerations. *Can. Anaesth. Soc. J*; **31:**541.

Shilbrolet S. *et al.* (1976). Heat stroke — a review. *Aviat. Space, Environ. Med*; **47:**280.

Walshaw M.J., Pearson M.G. (1984). Hypoxia in patients with acute hemiplegia. *Brit. Med. J*; **288:**15.

# CHAPTER 11

# Prolonged pain and palliative care

To act is so easy, to think is so hard.

*J.W. von Goethe*

## Introduction

There is a remarkable growth of pain relief clinics in which anaesthetists are involved and there are many textbooks on intractable pain, chronic pain and persistent pain relief. In these books the older patient features mostly in relation to 'terminal' pain care, for which ablation treatments are sometimes advocated, and the distressing conditions of thalamic, post-herpetic or phantom pains which are resistant to most treatments. There is, however, evidence of widespread suffering from pains which often older patients and their doctors accept as inevitable and untreatable, as if they are a consequence of ageing. In Northwick Park Hospital pain relief clinic one-third of the patients are over 65 years old, and nearly half of these over 75 years old. Any anaesthetist should be able to advise on pain management when requested to reduce this suffering.

Because of the changing psychology of ageing patients, the expression of pain can be limited and the evils which accompany the ageing condition can, to some extent, aggravate a painful condition. These evils include poverty, sickness, isolation and futility which only a new humane society could ameliorate. Occasionally a pain complaint is magnified by anxiety over another functional worry which the elderly are loath to declare, for example a minor stroke, reduced hearing or sight. The range of painful conditions commonly encountered in the elderly is different from that occurring in young people, and they benefit most from small amounts of multiple therapies applied with caution, except when cure is clear cut (Table 11.1).

**Table 11.1**

*Commoner chronic pain complaints in the elderly*

| Area | Causes | Comments |
|------|--------|----------|
| Head | Temporal arteritis | ESR required |
| | Transient ischaemic attack | Headaches are uncommon but often serious |
| | Stroke and thalmic pain | |
| | Depression | |
| Mouth | Dental decay | |
| | Stomal ulcers | |
| Face | Trigeminal neuralgia | Relatively uncommon (1–2%) |
| | Post-herpes zoster neuralgia | |
| Trunk | Post-herpes zoster neuralgia | |
| | Spine referral — musculoskeletal including cervical spondylosis | |
| | Spine or rib fractures | |
| | Postoperative wound neuralgia and nerve trapping | |
| | Heart neurasthenia | |
| Back | Osteoarthritis and porosis | |
| | Paget's disease | Pain not inevitable |
| | Cancer metastasis | Primary often not obvious |
| | Coccydynia | |
| Limbs | Vascular insufficiency | |
| | Restless legs | |
| | 'Silent' fractures | |
| | Poor feet care — calosis and nail deformity | |
| | Dystrophia and Sudeck's atrophy | |
| | Phantom and stump pains | |

## The pain entity

Pain is as undefinable as anxiety or fear but it may be accepted that it is 'what the patient says hurts'. Because these are 'complaining' patients, a considerable number will be emotionally disturbed and some will be aggressive in response to the failure of medical help. If the doctor's response to a patient's complaint, however irrational, is exasperation, then he or she is inadequate as that patient's adviser.

Treatment must be circumscribed in order to limit side-effects that may be more of a burden to the patient than the pain, which itself is rarely life threatening. While it is tempting for anaesthetists to concentrate on anatomical or biochemical concepts and obvious physical factors involved with pain, we must remember that the mechanism depends a great deal on the emotional and rational aspects. Indeed, the interplay may be such that a distinction is impossible and little is gained by trying to designate a pain as psychogenic or organic, imagined or genuine. Nevertheless it may be helpful to conjecture that a pain may be primarily psychological or physical in origin. Any chronic pain requires treatment of the patient in pain as much as of the pain itself. This requires attention to the whole patient rather than treating him or her as a repository of abnormalities treatable by technical means—an unfamiliar approach for anaesthetists.

## Drug therapy

Basic analgesics range from aspirin to morphine. Aspirin, paracetamol or non-steroidal anti-inflammatory drugs are valuable first-line drugs to use, with attention to simple methods of reducing pain.

Codeine is a useful weak opioid comparable in strength to many newer agonist and agonist–antagonist opioids. Morphine and other strong narcotics have common unwanted side-effects, including nausea, vomiting, drowsiness, dizziness, confusion, sweating, constipation, and depression. It is rarely helpful or justified to use strong narcotics for non-malignant pain.

Anxiolytics and antidepressants, with occasionally anti-epileptics, are supplementary drugs which may avoid escalation to more and stronger analgesics. The unusual use of these drugs should be explained to patients. A clear, practical, logical regimen should be prescribed which the aged can comply with and understand. It is easier to be familiar with all aspects of a few drugs (Table 11.2).

Combinations of drugs are rarely of benefit because the effective (or toxic) doses of each constituent cannot coincide in many patients. Placebo effect—that is, a beneficial result from a seemingly inactive agent—will be apparent in at least one-third of the patients one treats. This is a salutary thought and it must

**Table 11.2**
*Analgesics and Supplementary Drugs*

| Drug | Dose range (mg) | Comment |
| --- | --- | --- |
| *Antidepressants* | | |
| Amitriptyline | 10–50/12 h | Slow full effect |
| Mianserin | 20–100/12 h | Less anticholinergic effect |
| *Anticonvulsant* | | |
| Carbamazepine | 100–400/12 h | Slow full effect |
| *Analgesics* | | |
| Soluble aspirin | 600–1200/6 h | Dyspepsia and gastrointestinal bleeding |
| Paracetamol | 500–1000/6 h | Excess metabolite injures liver |
| Naproxen | 150–500/12 h | Mostly renal excreted |
| Codeine | 30–60/6 h | Depress bowel and cough |
| Oxycodone | 30–60/6 h | Special order suppositories (Boots) |
| Buprenorphine | 0.2–0.8/8 h | Nausea and dysphoria common |
| Morphine sulphate | 5–100/4 h | Frail old may get cumulation ill-effects |
| Morphine sulphate tabs (slow release) | 10–100/8 h | Less controllable than solution |
| Diamorphine | 1.5–50/4 h | Very soluble; storage hydrolysis |
| Phenazocine | 2.5–25/4 h | Least sedative |
| *Antinauseant* | | |
| Metoclopramide | 5–10/8 h | Extrapyramidal side-effects |
| Prochlorperazine | 5–10/8 h | Also tranquilliser |
| *Corticosteroid* | | |
| Prednisolone | 5–20/8 h | Helps appetite and well-being |
| *Sedatives* | | |
| Temazepam | 10–20 at night | Short acting |
| Diazepam | 2–10/12 h | Long action; muscle relaxant |
| *Stimulant* | | |
| Dexamphetamine | 2.5–5 mane | Assists analgesic |
| *Tranquilliser* | | |
| Methotrimeprazine | 25–50/12 h | Also analgesic |

be remembered that those who respond this way are not necessarily the most neurotic, but may often be stable and extrovert people. Indeed, with any agents which we believe are active, our expectation of success will be transmitted to a patient and be beneficial. In fact 20% of all medicines have no known pharmacological action and succeed only as placebos, as indeed may some physical treatments, for example acupuncture, manipulation and local injections.

## Blocks

Any anaesthetist should be able to undertake nerve blocks

on request, aided if need be by scrutiny of anatomy textbooks, skeleton, or other aids. Both the somatic and autonomic nerves can be blocked with good results either for a short or a relatively long period. Bupivacaine is now the longest-acting local anaesthetic (up to 12 hours), and 7.5% phenol in an aqueous solution or freezing of nerves may produce an effective block for up to 2 years. Apart from the resultant analgesia, blocks have the added advantage that they may cure the patient through abolition of a pain → spasm → immobilisation → pain cycle or by abolition of a set pattern of memorisation. Frequently, especially after repetition of a block, the physiological effect far outlasts the pharmacological duration. Electrical stimulation through coated needles or x-ray image intensification and indicator injections may be essential aids for the more complex blocks. Being familiar with a limited number of the techniques will be found to be most rewarding. Somatic paravertebral nerve block by the medial approach is simple and should be more frequently used.

Other peripheral blocks which anaesthetists do not often use are difficult. For instance, with a painful inoperable hip, block of the quadratus femoris branch of the sciatic and the obturator nerves may be used. The results of these blocks are equivocal, possibly dependent upon associated physiotherapy. The stellate ganglion and the lumbar sympathetic blocks are required frequently, but for the limbs intravenous regional sympathetic blockade with guanethidine is sometimes a simpler alternative.

Blocks that need investigating in the elderly are those used prophylactically in the case of phantom and herpes zoster pain. If before amputation or in the acute phase of herpes zoster pain is relieved for a period, it may be that subsequent problems could be reduced (see Chapter 10).

## Other methods

Transcutaneous electrical nerve stimulation is now widely employed. Its only adverse effect is an occasional dermal erythema through excess use. For its proper use in older patients, much education and instruction is needed; this may be best provided by a nurse experienced in the method. Different types of apparatus make the purchase decision critical, and a major concern should be the form of electrode which is most suitable, easily applied and maintained.

Acupuncture also has considerable vogue at present. It is crucial for the sceptical anaesthetist to realise that there may be considerable difference between acupuncture analgesia for surgery and acupuncture 'cure of disease.' The latter is so different and puzzling for conventionally trained doctors that only observation of its use by a medically trained person will enable them to apply it with the degree of conviction which is essential.

When it is thought that the benefit-against-cost equation is favourable, then neurosurgical operations such as rhizotomy, cordotomy or pituitary ablation or advanced psychotherapy may be required. Hypnotherapy can be helpful (using a tape recording which may be repeated on many occasions) to elderly patients who are more liable to have slow recognition of new ideas and need a greater time for contemplation.

Other non-conventional methods of manipulation and dietary adjustment can contribute in a holistic approach to a patient in pain. Such an approach also requires attention to the work, pleasure and spiritual activities of the patient which an amateur or professional psychologist can direct.

## Palliative care and cancer pain relief

Too often, when conventional medicine has no cure for a patient's condition, they are left to their own devices. As inevitably everyone must die of something, this is a very serious neglect. The hospice movement has arisen from a lack of provision of support in these circumstances, and their ideas and intentions to provide total care for such patients and their relatives should be applied widely. Education, liaison and practical action are required from a team of medical and lay helpers. Supportive members of staff should be organised so that they can mobilise all that is required for the patient and family to cope with their condition. Most families can cope with a patient at home when it is feasible medically. The commonest requests for help at home are for night nursing, housework, laundry and shopping. Psychiatrists, hospital and district nurses, general practitioners, physiotherapists, social workers, home helps, religious teachers and administrators all have roles in perfecting this service.

With advanced cancer, the common complaints in order of frequency are weakness, loss of appetite, pain, insomnia, depression, dyspnoea and nausea or vomiting. From a number of surveys, pain with cancer occurs in about 60% of patients, with 15% having pain which is difficult to control. Most pain is due to the tumour infiltration of bone, nerves or visceral organs. Some is a result of therapy or is coincidental, for example musculoskeletal pain and bedsores. For some types of pain drugs other than analgesics may be added for better control (Table 11.3).

**Table 11.3**
*Pain types and helpful additional drugs*

| Pain type | Helpful additional drugs |
| --- | --- |
| Bone pain | Aspirin or other NSAIDs |
| Nerve compression<br>Lymphoedema<br>Cerebral pressure increase | Corticosteroids and diuretics |
| Dysaesthesia or stabbing | Antidepressant or antiepileptic |
| Muscle spasm | Relaxants, e.g. baclofen |
| Tenesmus | Phenothiazine or rectal belladonna |
| Gastric 'pressure' | Metoclopramide or antacid |
| Infected ulcer | Antibiotic |

Drugs proscribed for cancer pain in the aged are methadone, pethidine, pentazocine and dextromoramide. If pain persists despite using an analgesic and other appropriate drugs and non-drug methods, regular morphine or diamorphine is required. The dose of morphine is arrived at by equating it with the potency of the failed drugs, adding extra and adjusting up by frequent review. It should be regarded as an emergency and the doctor must be readily available to advise until the patient is pain free in 2–3 days. Few patients need more than 100 mg morphine 4-hourly. If injection is required for any failure of administration or control, then continuous subcutaneous infusion with a syringe pump is preferable.

*Continuous narcotic subcutaneous infusion using syringe driver method*

1. The previous 24-hour oral morphine dose (or its equivalent) is calculated and one-third of that is given as diamorphine.
2. Dissolve the 24-hour dose in 10 ml saline in a syringe and load it onto the driver.
3. Connect the syringe to an extension tube with a fine needle attached and start the driver to fill the tube.
4. Insert the needle in the subcutaneous fat of the abdomen or chest and cover with a transparent dressing (Fig. 11.1).
5. Set the rate of the driver to discharge 10 ml in 24 hours. (Check syringe volume after 30 min.).
6. Recharge the syringe, adjusting the dose if necessary, every 24 hours.
7. Change and resite the needle every 1–3 weeks.

Segmental analgesic block may be provided by direct application of narcotics to receptors in the spinal cord dorsal horn cells. Continuous extradural or intrathecal drug is therefore being administered from external or percutaneous reservoir systems. Clinical studies have not yet proved the

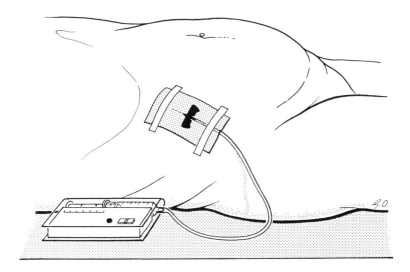

**Fig. 11.1** Diagram of the subcutaneous administration of drug into the abdominal wall with a syringe driving device.

value of these techniques or defined the complications fully. Late serious respiratory depression has been reported. Sudden respiratory depression has also occurred with narcotics given by other routes if pain is stopped by neural block.

Complaints other than of pain must be attended to as thoroughly as the pain. Also, review should be frequent as the pathological process may be modified by further radiation, hormone therapy or chemotherapy, or by surgery. These again require much circumspection in their application because they can also be the cause of complaints, including that of pain.

Restriction of necessary analgesics for fear of addiction is highly undesirable. Once begun, it is not inevitably essential to continue at a high dosage, because even extensive malignant destruction does not produce consistent or increasingly unbearable pain. It is quite unacceptable to use drastic ablation procedures with possible serious side-effects because the patients condition is terminal. A definition of 'terminal' is never exact, and in many instances patients with malignancies and other advanced conditions live for many years. The majority of patients want to know all about their condition and must be given time and opportunity to ask any questions, which should be answered truthfully and with extra kindness. Patients worry most about the means of dying, and less about the fact. A thoughtful surgeon has said, 'in treating cancer let us be realists: we may be able to cure only occasionally, but we can relieve often—and give hope always'. In all chronic pain care, such realism must be the basis of treatment.

**Further reading**

Editorial from the NIH (1979). Pain in the elderly—patterns of change with age. *J. Am. Med. Assoc*; **241**:2491.

Ellis H. (1981). Some aphorisms in cancer surgery. *Ann. Roy. Coll. Surg*; **61**:98.

Foley K. M. (1985). The treatment of cancer pain. *New. Eng. J. Med*; **313**:84.

Hanks G.W. *et al.* (1981). Unexpected complication of successful nerve block. Morphine induced respiratory depression precipitated by removal of severe pain. *Anaesth*; **36**(1):37.

Howard R.P. *et al.* (1981). Epidural morphine in teminal cancer. *Anaesth*; **36**:51.

Karko R. (1980). Age and morphine analgesia in cancer patients with post operative pain. *Clin. Pharm. Ther*; **28**:823.

Merksey H., Hester R.A. (1972). The treatment of chronic pain with psychotropic drugs. *Postgrad. Med. J*; **48**:594.

Neri M., Agazzani E. (1984). Ageing and right–left asymmetry in experimental pain measurement. *Pain*; **19**:43.

Pearse V., Robson P.J. (1980). Double blind crossover trial of meptazinol, pentazocine and placebo in the treatment of paid in the elderly. *Postgrad. Med. J*; **56**:474.

Poser C.M. (1976). Types of headache that affect the elderly. *Geriatrics*; **31**:103.

Rodstein M., Oei L. (1979). Cardiovascular side effects of long term therapy with tricyclic antidepressants in the aged. *J. Am. Geriatr. Soc*; **27**:231.

Rosenblatt R.M. *et al.* (1984). Tricyclic antidepressants in the treatment of depression and chronic pain. *Anesth. Analg*; **63**:1025.

Shumiather M.C. (1982). The good death maketh the bad life. *Ann. Roy. Col. Physicians Surg. Can*; **15**:216.

Trillin A.S. (1981). Of dragons and green peas—a cancer patient talks to doctors. *New Eng. J. Med*; **304**:699.

Twycross R.G., Fairfield S. (1982). Pain in far-advanced cancer. *Pain*; **14**:303.

Willcox J.C. *et al.* (1984). Prednisolone as an appetite stimulant in patients with cancer. *Brit. Med. J*; **288**:27.

# CHAPTER 12

# Resuscitation

> The lethal threshold falls until, in theory, the most trivial accident
> imaginable is the cause of death.
>
> *P.B. Medawar*

## Introduction

Prevention of the need for resuscitation of the elderly and aged is far more worthy than any heroic reanimation exercises. The old patient has had 'wear-and-tear', as well as perhaps having not been well looked after, so that chronic or acute illness can overwhelm more easily and preclude total recovery. The impact of chronic and subsequent acute illness can be disastrous, but with protection an old undiseased patient should defy a 'natural death'. Precipitation of the need for resuscitation within the orbit of the anaesthetist is likely to be most reduced if there is meticulous assessment, preparation and management of patients.

Universally in anaesthesia the precursors to cardiac arrest are obstructed airway or poor ventilation and hypovolaemia or drug misuse. Frequently these can be avoided or dealt with very early. If there is thought to be hypotension or some other drastic change in a patient's condition, one should immediately administer 100% oxygen briefly, while trying to assess the actual situation. There is far too frequently poor anticipation of problems, inattentiveness, or surprise at the rate at which a crisis arises, or excessive reliance is put upon pressor or antiarrhythmic drugs. At all times hypoxia should receive immediate prime attention together with assisted central venous blood return by the head-down and raised-legs posture of the patient. Any late or poor standard of care will be more dangerous because of the much reduced reserves of the old. With the greatest care we still face unpreventable incidences and the amount of resuscitation we should then undertake becomes questionable.

## Prognosis

This subject is part of the expanding controversy over medical ethics which causes anguish to many doctors. Older doctors were subject to the Hippocratic oath on qualifying. This included the statement 'I will follow the system which, according to my abilities and judgement, I consider for the benefit of my patients and abstain from whatever is deleterious or mischievous'. This should entail circumspect attempts at resuscitation for every arrest of breathing or pulse. The proscription of these attempts on the basis of age by edict, notification or whim is unsupportable. A brief application of mouth-to-mouth resuscitation or the use of a self-inflating bag for ventilation and closed cardiac massage are called for in all but the moribund *in extremis* patients.

Prolonged attempts at resuscitation are rarely indicated, but the very old have on occasion been totally returned to normality after such efforts. Rarely do difficult ethical decisions have to be made over who not to resuscitate or when to abandon efforts which are not immediately successful. This is because it is usual for the general state of the patient to have been well assessed and to be known to the medical attendants (Table 12.1).

**Table 12.1**

*Categories of old patients requiring cardiopulmonary resuscitation (CPR)*

| *No CPR* | *Difficult individual judgement of CPR* | *Compulsory CPR* |
|---|---|---|
| Chronically ill with progressive disease | Multiple cardiac arrests | Potentially well or unassessed subjects |
| Severely demented dependent subjects | Apnoea with good cardiac output | |
| Irreversible coma | Repeated epileptic seizures | |
| Dead on arrival | 'Terminal' carcinoma | |

In the case of older subjects there is no pressure from any quarter to make ethical decisions for the purpose of producing transplantable organs. The diagnosis of brain death may be complicated by the presence of metabolic, thermophilic or pharmacological abberations as well as by neurological dys-functions which are more common with ageing. If an apnoeic patient has been artificially ventilated and ultimate survival is not expected, it appears justified to remove any method of care which is clearly extraordinary and unnatural. If survival, even to a limited extent, is a possibility, it appears best to await the advent of cessation of circulation, which is rarely long delayed. Relatives should be fully and often informed of progress of events, with guarded prognosis at all times. This they will expect, but it is wrong to inflict unnecessary fears through precautionary pessimism. It is also wrong to be a prophet of doom and to predict an imminent death of which one cannot be certain.

Interoperatively, cardiac arrests can occur in fit young subjects in minor elective operations during the maintenance of anaesthesia by experienced anaesthetists. Because there are few fit survivors from such events, this indicates that observa-tion and monitoring or prompt resuscitation may be imperfect. In old patients failure can be due to underlying intractable disease, but it may also be more difficult to apply resuscitation efficiently.

It is generally agreed that prognosis in early severe shock is unreliable. However, the chance of long-term survival is obviously worse in older patients with underlying disease and when prolonged shock affects vital organs. When cardiac, respiratory or renal failure, jaundice or unconsciousness occur with shock in the elderly, survival is more rare.

Prediction of the outcome following myocardial infarction, hypovolaemia or septicaemia may be helped by cardiac output and/or pulmonary capillary pressure measurements. Peripheral skin temperature, combined with response to an intravascular infusion of fluid or dopamine, can be useful to predict future progress. Changes in arterial blood lactate levels or mixed venous blood oxygen tension, when available, may also give some evidence of progress. More crudely, in the case of trauma or burn, a scoring method for the severity of the injury has been found to give some guide to outcome.

It was claimed that with acute myocardial infarction mortal-ity was increased with age; however, with better care of coronary occlusion this is not evident. The complaints of old patients—arteriosclerosis, hypoxaemia, uraemia or septicaemia—all seriously worsen the outlook for quality of survival.

## Technique

External cardiac massage can only provide about one-third of the normal cardiac outflow of blood, much of this going to the brain. The kidney blood flow is markedly reduced during resuscitation and these organs are already jeopardised by ageing. To supply blood flow by direct pressure on the heart against the spine or by a general increase of intrathoracic pressure (the more recent explanation of the effectiveness of external cardiac massage), may be difficult with the usual inelastic chest wall of the older patient. The increased likelihood of chest wall injury during massage is obvious as are the obstacles of emphysema, barrel chest or marked vertebral deformity. Indeed, blood flow can be doubled by open massage, and this is indicated in many conditions common to older patients.

Difficult as it is to decide to open the chest, and however less practised and less prepared doctors are nowadays to perform this manoeuvre, it may be essential. For patients with severe mediastinal shift, cardiac tamponade, intrathoracic bleeding, flail chest, air embolism, pulmonary embolism, ruptured aortic aneurysm, or those resistant to defibrillation, open-chest cardiac massage is required. Some recent refinements—such as raising the legs or pressure on the abdomen, 50 per minute compression with 60% 'downtime', 1:3 ventilation-to-massage ratio, and massage on inspiration with higher peaks and some positive end-expiratory respiration or cough —are all in need of efficiency testing.

The state of expiration during defibrillation is said to be more propitious. Self-cough-induced cardiopulmonary resuscitation, automatic defibrillation, bretylium, therapeutic anaesthesia with barbiturates and relaxants are all experimental at present. Aspiration is a very common event in the old, even with a brief diminishing of the reflexes of protection. Indeed, choking is a common phenomenon, and if a solid object is blocking the glottis, it is not clear which is the best way of producing dislodgement. A strong blow on the back, abdominal epigastric thrust (Heimlich manoeuvre), chest thrusts or finger probing are all recommended by different authorities. All may fail, and endoscopy or cricothyrotomy be mandatory to overcome the obstruction.

When ventilation and cardiac output have been produced artificially, it is logical to complete the briefest treatment with a simple drug regimen. This requires the securing of an intravenous route and administration of a moderate dose of sodium bicarbonate while an electrocardiogram is being obtained. The findings of the trace should then initiate the appropriate treatment, as follows.

| | |
|---|---|
| Asystole | Adrenaline, calcium and dextrose |
| Bradycardia | Atropine and adrenaline |
| Ventricular tachycardia | Lignocaine and defibrillation |
| Ventricular fibrillation | Cardiac massage, adrenaline and defibrillation |

Current required for defibrillation can be standardised initially at 200 J, rising to 400 J depending on success. The relation of 10 J per year used in paediatrics is obviously inappropriate. If the patient has an implanted pacemaker, the defibrillator paddles should be placed at least 12 cm away from the pacemaker. The effect on circulation of intermittent positive pressure ventilation (IPPV) is now thought to be exceedingly complex. It is best to advocate the least mean intrathoracic pressure to produce an acceptable volume until the effect of various modifications of the form of IPPV may be clarified. The use of follow-up care for any consequent cerebral or renal hypoxic effects will depend on circumstances, but, it is logical if an immediate previous response to resuscitation has been obtained. Only when clear regimens are proved prospectively may we define their usefulness in each age group.

## Summary

If resuscitation is not prompt, a tragic damaged survivor may result and full success will rarely be achieved. Resuscitation attempts must not be pursued in old patients with progressing disease soon likely to lead to death. Conversely, resuscitation should not be withheld purely on a basis of age (however old) when the prearrest state of the patient is satisfactory, even if life expectency is short.

**Further reading**

Baker S.P. *et al.* (1974). The injury severity score—a method of describing patients with multiple injuries and evaluating emergency care. *J. Trauma*; **14**:187.

Campbell D. (1977). Immediate hospital care of the injured. *Brit. J. Anaesth*; **49**:673.

Champion H.R. *et al.* (1981). The trauma score. *Critical Care Med*; **9**:672.

Czer L.S.C., Shoemaker W.C. (1980). Myocardial shock in critically ill patients: response to whole blood transfusions as a prognostic measure. *Critical Care Med*; **8**:710.

Fusgen I., Summa J.D. (1978). How much sense is there in an attempt to resuscitate an aged person? *Gerontology*; **24**:37.

Gulati R.S. *et al.* (1983). Cardiopulmonary resuscitation of old people. *Lancet*; **ii**:267.

Lundberg G.D. (1983). Rationing human life. *J. Am. Med. Assoc*; **249**:2223.

Robertson G.S. (1983). Ethical dilemmas of brain failure in the elderly. *Brit. Med. J*; **287**:1775.

Skolimowski J. (1974). Successful resuscitation of a 94 year old patient. *Anaesth. Resusc. Int. Ther*; **2**(4):385.

Ruiz C.E. *et al.* (1979). Treatment of circulatory shock with dopamine. *J. Am. Med. Assoc*; **242**:165.

Vincent J.C. *et al.* (1981). Lactate metabolism during circulatory arrest. *Critical Care Med*; **9**:234.

Watts F.J.M., Nott M.B. (1977). The hazards of anaesthesia in the injured patient. *Brit. J. Anaesth*; **49**:707.

# CHAPTER 13

# Research

I seem to have been only like a boy playing on the seashore diverting myself and now and then finding a smoother pebble or a prettier shell than ordinary, whilst the great ocean of truth lay all undiscovered before me.

*A. Einstein*

The difficulties of carrying out research into older patients are comparable to those involving prisoners, children and the infirm. It is now widely accepted that informed consent is required. This is essential even if the treatment or procedure is common but irregular. Even regular therapeutic procedures with minimal risk may need extra drug administration or hospital admission, which for the old are major risks because drug reactions are more common and hospital stay potentially devastating. Investigation of new drugs rarely includes the study of their efficacy and safety in elderly patients. As drugs are predominantly used in these patients, this omission constitutes a serious neglect. Because of the older patients' difficulties in comprehension and their conservatism, they can be less available for research. However, because of the presence of multiple pathology in older patients, they may be exploited in studies—particularly in a free health service where older patients are inclined to feel grateful for their medical care and will comply with requests which may be quite unintelligible to them. When there is a risk it may be difficult to explain that the likelihood of its occurrence may be indefinable.

Dementia and mobility are subjects in urgent need of investigation in old patients. Anaesthetists could be involved in studies of both subjects, but there are particular concerns about this work. With dementia the patients with poor understanding are those who are required on research subjects, but consent of a relative for anything other than a possibly beneficial action would be unacceptable. Dementia may be related to abnormal neurotransmitter levels in the central nervous system, for example, diminished acetylcholine concentration, the number and sensitivity of receptors may be altered, and noradrenaline and serotonin levels reduced. Such changes may correlate with obvious changed responses to anaesthetics exhibited by these patients.

When studying the relief of pain in joints by nerve block as an aid to mobilisation, the procedure may be ineffective without the motivation of the patient, which we should aim to define more clearly. Also, although a block may improve mobility it may require manipulation for full benefit and be associated with adverse bowel action, urinary control or motor power of muscles more often than in young subjects.

Older patients may have inexplicable attitudes to what may appear to physicians to be routine studies. Thus in one city, intravenous sampling was acceptable but rectal examination rarely so, whereas potential subjects in another city approved of rectal examination but not of intravenous sampling. In some research projects multicentre planning can overcome the difficulties of collecting sufficient data in a short period of time. This is important with regard to the elderly because when obtaining data it will be found that the response rate is always lower than that for young patients. Broadly, it is said that older patients rarely respond to questionnaires containing more than five questions. Because the range of 'normality' broadens in the elderly, a larger sample will almost always be required for statistical decision.

When comparing mortality rates after a procedure, small age divisions of subjects must be employed, using the expected survival for each age group as a comparison, because any large age-range figures will not take account of 'natural death'. An urgent line of research concerns the capacity of the elderly to compensate for any demands of required surgery and anaesthesia. While we are rightly aware of the value of blood gas analysis as opposed to respiratory function tests, nevertheless neither assesses the reserve activity of the whole respiratory system. Studies of the physiological and biochemical responses to stresses of longevous patients could indicate what essentials have led to preservation of normality for such extended lives.

The major concerns in research of the old, particularly with regard to age changes, are the limitations and benefits of cross-sectional as opposed to longitudinal studies. Cross-sectional studies have been defined as concerning an observed difference at one point of time, and, of course, must take into consideration the many differences of the different age groups. There is little likelihood of studies following the medical state of a group of normal individuals from birth to death, or even from maturity to death. Sectional studies of population dominate the literature and different age groups will vary markedly in diet, voluntary activity, the drugs they have had recently and throughout their lives.

Each era has a different exposure to many aspects of environment which condition their 'healthy' state. For example, stimuli and training intellectually, personal and geographical pollution, domestic and national stresses will differ with each age group. These aspects may affect various organ systems differently. In the case of anaesthesia this is obvious in that the form of anaesthesia and perioperative care has changed immeasurably in recent decades.

Despite all the problems, including the financial requirement for longitudinal studies, it is to be hoped that with the expansion of the elderly population the government's previous 'cost-effective' plans will be changed so that a reasonable proportion of research money will be assigned to this major part of medical care. Anaesthetists should indicate their realisation of the need to expand their knowledge about older patients by actively encouraging their own and cooperative workers of this nature.

It should be obvious from the rest of this book that the number of indisputable facts known about anaesthesia in older patients is very limited. It is of interest that the proposed requirements for all new drugs in anaesthesia are those which would most benefit the older patient, for example short-acting and rapidly disposed agents. Every anaesthetist realises that general anaesthesia affects old and young patients differently. If these differences could be studied in detail, it is conceivable that the results would further our understanding of the mechanism of the state of anaesthesia.

Also it is unclear whether the impaired immune state of elderly patients is related to their sensitivity to infection. Perhaps if anaesthesia's effect on immune responses were explored deeply, it would be enlightening. Similarly, an understanding of the interaction of vitamin $B_{12}$ and nitrous oxide might shed light on other anaesthetic or haematological matters. Every aspect of an anaesthetist's clinical work with the elderly patient is in need of some research (Table 13.1).

## Table 13.1

*Areas of anaesthesia research: some projects for exploration in patients aged 60–75 and 75–90*

*Preoperatively*
Assessment non-invasively with many new and old modified techniques
Assessment of autonomic competence
Assessment of cerebral state
Preplanned progressive treatment, financial and medical studies
Fitness training effects
Nutritional adjustment

*General anaesthesia*
Define and refine loss of consciousness
Preoxygenation relationship to lung stage
Control of dangerous reflexes
Heat balance
Ventilation control ($Paco_2$ and cerebral flow)
Control of relaxants and their antidotes

*Local anaesthesia*
Practical nerve blocks
Ideal sedation supplementation
Drug concentration requirement for differential block
Extension of block duration
Spinal block objective level assessments
Vasodilation control or management

*Postoperatively*
Mini tracheostomy toilet usage
Preplanned ventilation control
Mandatory minute volume weaning
Active limitation of confusion

*Intensive therapy*
Resuscitation; gauge success of routine simple techniques plus home care tuition
Treatment: refine invasive and non-invasive monitoring and relate value to complications

*Pain relief*
Non-malignant: predict subjects and assess social factors
Malignant: collect data of amount and natural history outcome

**Further reading**

Bernstein J.E., Nelson F.K. (1975). Medical experimentation in the elderly. *J. Am. Geriatr. Soc*; **23**:3.

Das S.K. *et al.* (1979). Geriatric medicine: model for computer oriented research analysis. *J. Am. Geriatr. Soc*; **1**:27.

Denham M.J. (1984). The ethics of research in the elderly. *Age & Ageing*; **13**:321.

Holliday R. (1984). The ageing process is a key problem in biomedical research. *Lancet*; **2**:1386.

Ratzan R.M. (1980). Being old makes you different! The ethics of research with elderly subjects. *Hastings Center Rep*; **10**:32.

Reich W. T. *et al.* (1978). Ethical issues in research involving elderly subjects. *Gerontologist*; **18**: 326.

Wilcock G.K. (1979). Use of a self-administered postal questionnaire when screening for health problems in the elderly. *Gerontology*; **25**:345.

# Theories of ageing

After sexual maturity and the end of growth we accumulate physiological decrements that increase the likelihood of dying. The effect of this is to clear away members of each succeeding generation. In ageing cultured human cells, 125 functional changes have been found to date. These occur in DNA, RNA, enzymes, cell-cycle genetics, lipids, carbohydrate and protein synthesis, degradation, morphology and karyology. When human embryonic tissue is cultured, 50 population doublings are usually the limit. Many basic sciences combined with clinical experience produce many theories of ageing. The following are those which have morphological support at present.

1. *Autoimmunity.* Mutation causes autoantigens of cytoplasm or nuclei to form. The surrounding body then reacts to the affected cells to make them malfunction, as in arthritis and diabetes.

2. *Collagen deposit.* Fibrosis is widespread, especially in endocrine, reproductive and muscle structure, possibly replacing degenerating tissue.

3. *Wear-and-tear.* This is indicated by the rate of metabolic energy expenditure which determines the life span. Perhaps pigment deposits in brain, muscle and liver show cell wear without repair.

4. *Chromosomal theory.* The increase of aberrations in the mitotic figures of old cells may produce malfunction. The rate of increase can correlate with the life span.

5. *Gene mutation.* Each species has its longevity value, i.e. there appears to be a genetic basis for life span. Because there is spontaneous somatic mutation, altered structure causes malfunction—senility. It could be that somatic mutation leads to chromosomal abnormality with autoimmune consequences, including collagen and pigment deposition or degeneration, thus linking these theories and, incidentally, biological and pathological ageing.

# Laboratory investigations

It is common to screen ill elderly patients biochemically. The levels found most helpful are those of calcium, alkaline phosphatase, albumin, serum $T_4$ and $T_3$ uptake, random blood sugar, urea and electrolytes. Some values of substances undoubtedly change with ageing, for example the 'normal' urea and creatinine levels are higher in an old person, but still indicate poorer renal function, due to ageing or disease. This altered renal function may also affect uric acid, phosphate, electrolytes and calcium levels. Conversely, the albumin level is lower with ageing and changes in serum proteins may affect the level of substances substantially bound to proteins, for example calcium, thyroid hormone or serum iron. Carrier proteins tend to fall even lower in ill patients and cause an equally marked reduction of the substance carried. Unrecognised illness, such as Paget's disease or osteomalacia, may be the explanation of the commonly observed increase in alkaline phosphatase levels.

Changes in sex steroids and anabolic steroids are more complex in their effect on thyroid function tests and calcium or phosphorous levels. Also, very common routine therapies, for example with diuretics, may affect the sodium and potassium levels by means of increased renal loss.

*Changes in levels of substances with ageing*
   *1. Levels of substances raised in old age.*
Alkaline phosphatase, globulin, urea, creatinine, uric acid, cholesterol, calcium (in women),

$$\text{ESR (men } \frac{\text{age}}{2}, \text{ women } \frac{\text{age} + 10}{2} \text{ mm/1st h)}$$

   *2. Levels of substances decreased in old age.*
Albumin, phosphate (in men), serum $T_3$, serum iron, total iron-binding capacity (TIBC), white blood cell count (WBC).

3. *Levels of substances unchanged in old age.*
Serum sodium, serum potassium, serum chloride, serum bicarbonate, magnesium, bilirubin, acid phosphatase, serum $T_4$.

*Biochemical values which differ from those of middle age*

| | |
|---|---|
| Calcium | 2.2–2.7 mmol/l (8.5–11.5 mg/100 ml) |
| Phosphate | 0.7–1.5 mmol/l (2.1–4.6 mg/100 ml) |
| Urea | 4–10 mmol/l (22–60 mg/100 ml) |
| Creatinine | 40–170 μmol/l (0.4–1.8 mg/100 ml) |
| Protein | 60–80 g/l (6–8 g/100 ml) |
| Albumin | 33–49 g/l (3.3–4.9 g/100 ml) |
| Globulin | 22–42 g/l (2.2–4.2 g/100 ml) |
| Cholesterol | 4–11 μmol/1 (180–435 mg/100 ml) |
| Alkaline phosphatase | <25 KAU (<150 i.u./1) |

*Haematological values which differ from those of middle age*

| | |
|---|---|
| Haemoglobin | 11.5–12 g/dl |
| Leucocytes (WBC) | 3000–8500/mm$^3$ |
| Lymphocytes | 700–3000/mm$^3$ |
| Serum folate | >1.5 μg/1 |
| Serum iron | >9 μmol/l (750 μg/100 ml) |
| TIBC | 47–72 μmol/l (240–400 μg/100 ml) |

# Surgical mortality

In a British surgical ward about one-third of all admissions are aged 65 or over. More than one-third are emergency admissions and about half of them are operated upon. Older patients, on the whole, stay twice as long in hospital, primarily due to postoperative morbidity, 10% of which is due to residual malignancy. It has been suggested that a different system of auditing surgical mortality is needed to take account of the potential viability of patients, the medical or surgical causes of death, and which patients are operated upon. However, only the last-mentioned are clearly definable. In one such assessment the overall mortality for patients aged 65–75 years old was 9.9%, and for those over 75 years 20.9%, whereas if non-viable patients were excluded the mortality rates were 1.4% and 6.6%, respectively. The better results in viable patients could encourage the optimistic approach required. Although less than one-fifth of all operations involve the elderly, they account for over half of the mortality for all ages. Expressed differently, it is stated that patients aged over 75 years comprise only 5% of the surgical population, but amongst those who die within 6 days of operation this proportion is increased tenfold. The overall mortality for the hospital stay is approximately 5% in the majority of published results.

Of course the type of operation undertaken is important as a larger proportion of the elderly undergo major operations in emergency conditions than at other ages. The specific operation is also important: whereas in eye surgery only 1 death per 1000 operations is reported, up to one-third of all midthigh amputations are followed by death. Long-term follow-up will produce high mortality figures but they appear not to be significantly higher than expected for the age group involved. The most important factor in the production of primary mortality figures is the state of the patient at operation (this may apply to any age). Patients with dementia, congestive cardiac failure, ischaemic heart disease, poor renal function and diabetes all have a raised mortality rate for elective operations, and this is doubled for emergency undertakings. However, if there is no serious preoperative disease, there is not much difference in the mortality from the average for all ages, except in the very aged.

### Further reading

Aubrey U. *et al.* (1965). Factors affecting survival of the geriatric patient after major surgery. *Can. Anaesth. Soc. J*; **12**(5):510.

Denny J. L., Denson J. S. (1972). Risks of surgery in patients over 90. *Geriatrics*; **27**:115.

Djokovic J.L., Hedley-Whyte J. (1979). Prediction of outcome of surgery and anaesthesia in patients over 80. *J. Am. Med. Assoc*; **242**(21):2301.

Gallaunaugh S.C. *et al.* (1976). Regional survey of femoral head fractures. *Brit. Med. J*; **2**:1496.

Kathic M. R. (1985). Surgery in centenarians. *J. Am. Med. Assoc*; **253**:3139.

Linn B.S. *et al.* (1982). Evaluation of results of surgical procedures in the elderly. *Ann. Surg*; **195**:90.

Lewin I. *et al.* (1971). Physical class and physiologic status in the prediction of operative mortality in the aged sick. *Ann. Surg*; **174**:217.

Mohr D.N. (1983). Estimation of surgical risk in the elderly: a correlative review. *J. Am. Geriatr. Soc*; **31**:99.

Palmberg S., Hirsjarvi E. (1979). Mortality in geriatric surgery. With special reference to the type of surgery, anaesthesia, complicating diseases, and prophylaxis of thrombosis. *Gerontology*; **25**(2):103.

Santos A.L., Gelperin A. (1975). Surgical mortality in the elderly. *J. Am. Geriatr. Soc*; **23**:42.

Seymour D.G., Pringle R. (1982). A new method of auditing surgical mortality rates — application to a group of elderly surgical patients. *Brit. Med. J*; **284**:1539.

Stevens K.M., Aldrete J.A. (1969). Anesthesia factors affecting surgical morbidity and mortality in the elderly male. *J. Am. Geriatr. Soc*; **17**(7):659.

Young H.D. *et al.* (1971). Major abdominal surgery in the elderly: a review of 172 consecutive patients. *Can. J. Surg*; **14**:324.

Ziffren S.E. (1979). Comparison of mortality rates of various surgical operations according to age group. *J. Am. Geriatr. Soc*; **27**:433.

# Mental assessment of patients

Mental testing is imprecise, especially when undertaken by those not familiar with the process. It should not be considered a diagnostic test but merely a screening device in which those who perform fairly well are unlikely to have any serious dementing condition. Normal ageing will give changes in the results of such tests and it must be recognised that while speed and flexibility will be lost, this can be counteracted by experience, wisdom and control.

A rapid progressive decrease in a mental test score over a period of months is serious, but a gradual decline is unlikely to be so. It is important to ensure that aphasia, agnosia or dyspraxia is not the cause of a poor performance. Depressed patients may also score badly and complain of memory failure so commonly that it has been called 'pseudodementia'.

The simpler tests that can be administered by the unskilled will only detect fairly advance changes. Simple memory information type questions can be used (see questionnaire) and these should be appropriate for the particular population being questioned.

### Modified Tooting Bec Questionnaire

*Introduction to patient*
'Some people as they get older often tend to forget things. I should like to ask you some questions to see how well you remember things which have happened recently in the past.'

(a) What is your name?

(b) How old are you?

(c) Are you married?

(d) What was your work? (Ask women about their work before marriage)

(e)  What year is it?

(f)  What is the name of this hospital? (If not known, inform)

(g)  I am going to tell you an address, and I want you to remember it: 74 Columbia Road

(h)  What year did the Second World War start? and finish?

(i)  Who was the Prime Minister at the end of the war?
                                        the beginning of the war?

(j)  Who is the Prime Minister now?

(k)  What is the name of the queen?

(l)  What is the name of her eldest son?

(m) Where is Belfast?

(n)  What is happening there now?

(o)  Now tell me the name of the hospital again?

(p)  Tell me the address that I told you.

*Conditions in which mental test questionnaires are inapplicable*

- *Dysphasia*
- *Deafness*
- *Depression*
- *Disturbed consciousness*
- *Native language difficulties*
- *Severe illness, making the patient unable to cooperate*

*Source:* Denham M.J., Jefferys P.M. (1978). *Medicine*; **1**:1.

If less than half of the questions can be answered correctly, the patient may have cerebral pathology, and a retest lower score may indicate permanent impairment whereas improvement will suggest that further expert testing should be undertaken together with an extended symptom and sign assessment. Other short tests concentrating on memory and fluency have utilised the naming of as many words beginning with a certain letter in 1 minute or naming as many items as can be recalled in each of four categories or sets, for example colours, animals, fruits or towns. With the latter, if 10 items are accepted as the requirement for each set, no patient who scores over 25 could be considered to have dementia.

Visual–motor performance can be measured by joining together with a line 25 numbers scattered over a page, or by joining numbers and letters alternatively in sequence. Unfortunately these tests have rarely been studied in patients with functional psychiatric disorders. Although by no means proving organic disease, they should stimulate more evaluation if they are done poorly because the poor performance can reflect a great variety of causes other than organic disease.

More extensive testing of the overall brain function, as undertaken by clinical psychologists, has principally developed from school intelligence tests. That most widely known is the Wechsler Adult Intelligence Scale (WAIS) which has been standardised for a large age range (Table D.1). It is time consuming and requires training for administration, scoring and interpretation. It consists of 11 subtests, 6 of which are classified as verbal and 5 as performance. The full IQ scale is derived from the verbal and performance scores. In some instances the separation of the verbal and performance results may be important because in normal subjects they are rarely more than a few points apart.

**Table D.1**
*The Wechsler Adult Intelligence Scale (related to age)*

| Age (years) | Verbal score | Performance score | Normal IQ for varying age |
|---|---|---|---|
| 30 | 60 | 50 | 100 |
| 60 | 56 | 37 | Decrement of 7% and 26% |
| 74 | 44 | 25 | Decrement of 27% and 50% |

With increased age the increasing percentage of the population experiencing decreased performance on testing inevitably means that an elderly patient can have considerable impairment of function (compared with that of early years) with an IQ within the normal range. Although the test is valuable, it must be recognised that false negatives should be expected and that false positives can occur.

The Wechsler memory scale assesses not only general function but also some discretionary function. There are many other tests (particularly in the USA) for measuring discrete qualities including those for abstraction, reasoning and problem solving, visual or motor performance, language function and personality. For the last-mentioned the most commonly used is the Minnesota Multiphasic Personality Inventory (MMPI) which is a true/false questionnaire of several hundred items requiring computer interpretation. Whereas even this complex test may indicate organic dysfunction, it does not measure it directly or establish a diagnosis, it is merely like all other psychological tests, an aid to clinical evaluation lacking specificity and is often given unwarranted validity.

.

## APPENDIX E

# Indices

### 1. *Cardiac Risk*

| Points | Factors |
|---|---|
| 11 | Third heart sound—jugular venous distension (congestive failure) |
| 7 | Important arrhythmia |
| 7 | >5 premature ventricular (beats/min) |
| 10 | Myocardial infarction <6/12 previously |
| 3 | Aortic stenosis |
| 5 | Older than 70 years |
| 3 | Poor medical condition |
| | $Pao_2$ <60 mmHg (8 kPa) |
| | $Paco_2$ >50 mmHg (6.7 kPa) |
| | Potassium <3 mmol/l |
| | Bicarbonate <20 mmol/l |
| | Serum urea >8 mmol/l |
| | Bedridden—creatinine increase, transaminase increase (liver disease) |
| 3 | Abdominal or chest operation |
| 4 | Emergency operation |

| | | |
|---|---|---|
| Class 1 | Score | 0–5 |
| Class 2 | | 6–12 |
| Class 3 | | 13–25 |
| Class 4 | | 26+ |

From Goldman *et al.* (1977). Multifactorial index of cardiac risk in non-cardiac surgical procedures. *New Engl. J. Med*; **297**:845.

### 2. *Exercise tolerance (New York Heart Association)*

| Class | Exercise tolerance |
|---|---|
| 1 | No limit of physical activity |
| 2 | Ordinary daily activity → fatigue, palpitation, dyspnoea |
| 3 | Exertion of less than daily activity → fatigue, palpitation, dyspnoea |
| 4 | Symptoms at rest |

*Note.* For old patients, activity is limited, dyspnoea is insidious and associates are incapacitated 'norms'.

## 3.   Score of risk of developing pressure sores

| Score | General physical condition | Mental state | Activity | Mobility | Incontinence |
|---|---|---|---|---|---|
| 4 | Good | Alert | Ambulant | Full | None |
| 3 | Fair | Apathetic | Walks with help | Slightly limited | Occasional |
| 2 | Poor | Confused | Chairbound | Very limited | Usually urine |
| 1 | Very bad | Stuperose | Bedfast | Immobile | Doubly |

Maximum score = 20; < 14 = at risk; < 12 = great risk.

From Norton D. *et al.* (1976). *An Investigation of Geriatric Nursing Problems in Hospital.* London: The National Company for the Care of Old People.

## 4.   Pulse rate correlation with American Society of Anesthesiologists (ASA) score

| ASA | Pulse rate (beats/min) | Pulse rate/maximum pulse rate* (beats/min) |
|---|---|---|
| 1 | 40–90 | 0.25–0.45 |
| 2 | 90–120 | 0.45–0.60 |
| 3 | 120–150 | 0.60–0.75 |
| 4 | 150–180 | 0.75–0.90 |
| 5 | >180 | >0.90 |

*Maximum pulse rate = 220 − age (years).

## 5.   Post-anaesthetic recovery score

|  | Score |
|---|---|
| *Activity* | |
| Number of extremities able to move voluntarily or on command | |
| 4 | 2 |
| 2 | 1 |
| 0 | 0 |
| *Respiration* | |
| Able to breathe deeply or cough freely | 2 |
| Dyspnoea or limited breathing | 1 |
| Apnoea | 0 |
| *Circulation* | |
| BP ± 30% preop. level | 2 |
| BP ± 30–50% preop. level | 1 |
| BP ± 50% preop. level | 0 |

*5 continued*

|  | *Score* |
|---|---|
| *Consciousness* | |
| Fully awake | 2 |
| Arousable on calling | 1 |
| Not responding | 0 |
| *Colour* | |
| Pink | 2 |
| Pale, dusky, blotchy | 1 |
| Cyanotic | 0 |

Score < 7 needs continued observation. Also observe temperature, vomiting and pain control.

From Aldrete J., Kroulik D. (1970). A postoperative recovery score. *Anesth. Analg*; **49**:924.

# General bibliography

Chappel W.A. *et al.* (1982). Anaesthesia and the elderly. *S. Afr. Med. J*; **62**:399.

Coulthard S.W., Millar R.W. (1981). Anesthesia for the elderly and debilitated patient. *Otolaryngol. Clin. N. Am*; **14**:715.

Dobson M.E. (1984). Anaesthesia in the elderly. *In Clinical Pharmacology and Drug Treatment in the Elderly* (O'Malley K., ed.) p. 196. Edinburgh: Churchill Livingstone.

Dundee J.W. (1979). Response to anaesthetic drugs in the elderly. In *Drugs and the Elderly* (Crooks J., Stevenson I.H., eds.) p. 179 London: Macmillan.

Ellison N. (1975). Problems in geriatric anesthesia. *Surg. Clin. N. Am*; **55(4)**:929.

Evans T.I. (1973). The physiological basis of geriatric general anaesthesia. *Anaesth. Int. Care*; **1**:319.

Evans T.I. (1977). Problems in general anaesthesia. Geriatrics. *Aust. Fam. Physician*; **6(4)**:339.

Gordon J.L. (1977). Planning a safe anesthesia for the elderly patient. *Geriatr*; **32**:69.

Griffith H.R. (1966). Problems in anaesthesiology for the aged. *Can. Anaesth. Soc. J*; **13**:14.

Krechel S.W.,ed. (1984). *Anesthesia and the Geriatric Patient.* London: Grune and Stratton.

Lesnick G.J., Weiss M.R. (1980). Surgery in the elderly: attitudes and facts. *Mt. Sinai J. Med. (N.Y.)*; **47(2)**:208.

Miller R. *et al.* (1977). Anesthesia for patients aged over 90 years. *N.Y. State J. Med*; **77**:1421.

Miller R.D., ed. (1981). Anesthesia for the elderly. In *Anesthesia*, Vol. 2. p. 1231. New York: Churchill Livingstone.

Parkhouse J. (1978). Anaesthesia in old age. In *Text Book of Geriatric Medicine and Gerontology*, 2nd edn. (Brocklehurst J.C., ed.) p. 731. Edinburgh: Churchill Livingstone.

Powell K. (1979). Anaesthesia for the aged. In *Surgical Problems in the Aged*. (Vowles K.D.J., ed.) p. 30. Bristol: John Wright.

Roberts M.T. (1976). Anaesthesia for the geriatric patient. *Drugs*; **11**:220.

Robertson J.D. (1980). Anaesthesia and the geriatric patient. In *General Anaesthesia*, 2nd edn, Vol. 2 (Gray J.C., Nunn J.F., Utting J.E., eds.) p. 1433. London: Butterworth.

Scott D.L. (1961). Anaesthetic experiences in 1300 major geriatric operations. *Brit. J. Anaesth*; **33**:345.

Vowles K.D.J. (1981). Surgical traps in the elderly. *Brit. J. Hosp. Med*; **16**:454.

Warren M.W. (1943). Care of chronic sick. A case for treating chronic sick in blocks in a general hospital. *Brit. Med. J*; **1**:822.

White D.G. (1980). Anaesthesia in old age. *Brit. J. Hosp. Med*; **24**:145.

## Sources of figures not in further reading references

Fig. 1.1 Freis J. F. (1980). Ageing, natural death and compression of morbidity. *New Eng. J. Med*; **303**:130.

Figs. 1.4 and 1.13 Hershey D., Wang H. H. (1980). *A New Age Scale for Humans*. Lexington: Lexington Books.

Fig. 1.8 Hodkinson H. M. (1983). Biochemical changes in old age. *Med. Int*; **1**:1701.

Fig. 1.10 Goldman R. (1970). Speculations on vascular changes with age. *J. Am. Geriatric Soc*; **18**:765.

Fig. 2.2 *Growing Older* (1981). HMSO. London:

Fig. 2.3 Overstall P. W. *et al.* (1977). Falls in the elderly related to postural imbalance. *Brit. Med. J*; **1**:261.

Fig. 3.2 Renray Rollers, Renray Ltd., Winsford, Cheshire CW7 3RB.

Fig. 4.2 MRC Working Party (1981). Long term domicillary oxygen therapy in chronic hypoxic cor-pulmonale complicating chronic bronchitis and emphysema. *Lancet*; **1**:681.

  Fletcher C., Peto R. (1977). The natural history of chronic air flow obstruction. *Brit. Med. J*; **1**:1645.

Fig. 5.8 Tachibana N. (1975). Somatosensory evoked potentials. *Int. Anesthesiol. Clin*; **13**:1.

# Index